SAQs for Dentistry
Third Edition

SAQs for Dentistry
Third Edition

Kathleen F M Fan PhD, MBBS, BDS, FDSRCS (Eng), FRCS (Ed), FRCS (OMFS)
Consultant Oral and Maxillofacial Surgeon,
Honorary Senior Lecturer
King's College Hospital, London

Judith Jones BDS, MSc, FDSRCS (Eng), PhD, FDS (OS), FHEA
Reader / Honorary Consultant, Department of Oral and Maxillofacial Surgery, Queen Mary University of London, Barts and the London School of Medicine and Dentistry, Institute of Dentistry

Pastes⁺

© 2015 Pastest Ltd

Egerton Court

Parkgate Estate
Knutsford
Cheshire
WA16 8DX

Telephone: 01565 752000

First Published 2007
Second Edition Published 2012
Third Edition Published 2015

ISBN: 9781905635993
A catalogue record for this book is available from the British Library.

Pastest Online Revision, Books and Courses

Pastest provides online revision, books and courses to help medical students and doctors maximise their personal performance in critical exams and tests. Our in-depth understanding is based on over 40 years' experience and the feedback of recent exam candidates.

Resources are available for:
Medical school applicants and undergraduates, MRCP, MRCS, MRCPCH, DCH, GPST, MRCGP, FRCA, Dentistry, Interview Skills, and USMLE Step 1.

For further details contact:
Tel: 01565 752000   Fax: 01565 650264
www.pastest.co.uk   enquiries@pastest.co.uk

Text prepared in the UK by Carnegie Book Production, Lancaster
Printed and bound in the UK by Page Bros Ltd, Norwich

Contents

List of Contributors

Dr A W Barrett BDS MSc PhD FDS RCS (Ed & Eng) FRCPath
Consultant Oral Pathologist
Queen Victoria Hospital
East Grinstead

Julia Costello BDS MSc
Clinical Demonstrator Department of Periodontology
Guy's Hospital,
Kings College London

Richard Jones BDS MSc FDSRCS M. Orth.RCS
Specialist Orthodontic Practitioner
Total Orthodontic Ltd
Sussex

Dr Virginia J Kingsmill PhD BDS FDSRCS
Lecturer
Department of Conservative Dentistry
Barts and The London Queen Mary School of Medicine and Dentistry

Sanjeev Sood BDS MFDS RCSEd MDent ChFDS
Senior Specialist Teacher/Honorary Consultant in Paediatric Dentistry
King's College Dental Institute, London

Professor Saman Warnakulasuriya
Professor of Oral Medicine
King's College, London

Introduction

Methods of examining and assessing students have changed over recent years. Traditional essay writing is not as popular as it once was and is often replaced with short answer questions (SAQs). The advantage of SAQs over essays is that they allow a wider range of topics to be examined in a single paper, and the marking is often more objective. They test knowledge recall as well as application of knowledge and understanding of principles.

The questions themselves can take a variety of formats, for example writing notes on a subject, filling in blanks in a paragraph, selecting the appropriate response from a list or one-line answers. Questions often have many inter-related parts. SAQs are usually not negatively marked so it is worth attempting all questions. In most examinations the questions usually have equal marks allocated to them unless otherwise stated. This often gives you a clue as to how much detail is expected in an answer for a particular question. This book does not include a marking scheme, but most questions ask for a particular number of responses.

The aim of the book is to help candidates assess their knowledge and identify the areas where they need to read more, as well as providing valuable examination practice. It is intended to be used as a revision aid for students taking the undergraduate or postgraduate examinations in dentistry, such as BDS, ORE, MJDF and MFDS. Common and popular topics have been covered but it was not possible to cover the entire scope of dentistry comprehensively in the book! We hope that you will find this book to be helpful and easy to use.

Good luck for the forthcoming exams.

Kathleen Fan and Judith Jones

1
Child Dental Health and Orthodontics

1.1 An 8-year-old boy attends your practice with his mother. He is medically fit and well, and has accepted dental treatment with a local anaesthetic on a previous occasion. Their main concern is the slight sensitivity that he is having from his back teeth and some white marks on his front teeth. On examination you diagnose molar incisor hypomineralisation (MIH).

(a) What is MIH?

(b) Clinically, you note: mild enamel opacities with minimal enamel breakdown on his mandibular first permanent molars, and mild enamel opacities without enamel breakdown on his maxillary first permanent molars. How would you manage the permanent posterior molars?

Answer 1.1

(a) MIH is a developmentally derived dental defect that involves hypomineralisation of one to four first permanent molars (FPMs), frequently associated with similarly affected permanent incisors (Weerheijm et al, 2003).

(b)

- Prevention: (high-risk) fluoridated toothpaste ≥1350 ppm fluoride, fissure seal permanent molars with resin sealant, apply fluoride varnish to teeth three to four times yearly (2.2% F⁻), prescribe daily fluoride rinse, investigate diet and assist adoption of good dietary practice

- Stabilisation: you may wish to stabilise the dentition with a glass ionomer cement (GIC); consider orthodontic referral to discuss long-term plans for retention of first permanent molars and discuss extractions at appropriate age/stage of dental development

- Sensitivity: fluoride (mouth wash, varnish), casein (phosphopeptide—amorphous calcium phosphate, CPP-ACP) tooth mousse, seal and bond

- May need to use nitrous oxide sedation to help with compliance because teeth may be tricky to anaesthetise, or consider the use of alternative local anaesthetic (eg articaine infiltration)

- Fissure sealants (FSs) are useful for molars with mild defects and without breakdown

- Restorations:

  - Amalgam is a non-adhesive material and its use is not indicated

  - Restorations with GIC and resin-modified GIC are not recommended in stress-bearing areas of FPMs, and they can be used only as an intermediate approach until a definite restoration has been placed

  - Definitive restoration should be carried out using local anaesthetic and under rubber dam isolation. Restoration of choice is a composite resin

Weerheijm KL, Duggal M, Mejare I, Papagiannoulis L, Koch G, Martens LC, et al. Judgement criteria for molar incisor hypomineralization (MIH) in epidemiologic studies: a summary of the European meeting on MIH held in Athens, 2003. *Eur J Paediatr Dent* 2003; **4**:110–113.

1.2 (a) Maxillary canines are commonly impacted. What signs might a general dental practitioner see in a patient's mouth that would make them suspicious that a maxillary canine was impacted in a 13-year-old patient?

(b) What special investigations would be warranted?

(c) In what circumstances would you consider the surgical removal of an impacted canine tooth?

(d) In what circumstances would you consider leaving the impacted canine where it is?

Answer 1.2

(a)

- Absence of maxillary canine in the appropriate position in the mouth
- Absence of a canine bulge palpable in the buccal sulcus
- Deciduous upper canine still in place and firm
- Protrusion of the lateral incisor
- Other associated dental anomalies — hypodontia, malformed teeth, delayed eruption of teeth, enamel hypoplasia

(b) In the first instance a radiograph should be taken to determine whether the tooth is present. An upper standard occlusal view or a periapical view should show the tooth, or if necessary a dental tomograph could be taken. If only one view is taken and a tooth is visible then a further radiograph in another plane can be taken to allow more accurate localisation of the tooth. A cone beam CT (CBCT) of the impacted canine and adjacent teeth is often helpful to provide further information about their relationship and any associated pathology, eg resorption of the adjacent tooth, that may impact on the treatment plan.

(c)

- When the tooth shows pathology associated with it, for example a dentigerous cyst or root resorption.
- When there is evidence of root resorption of adjacent teeth which appears to be caused by the impacted canine tooth.
- Where a patient is having orthodontic treatment to align the adjacent teeth to create an arch form without utilising the canine and the canine is thought to be in the way of planned orthodontic tooth movement.
- If the patient chooses the option of an implant to replace the canine and avoid the need for extended orthodontic treatment.

(d)

- Where there is no pathology associated with the impacted canine.
- The patient is not having orthodontic treatment that requires its removal.

- There is a risk of damaging the adjacent teeth/tooth by removing it.

- When a patient declines to have it removed even though there are indications to remove it.

- Where there are contraindications in the medical history to removal of the tooth.

1.3 (a) What are the various components of a removable orthodontic appliance and what function does each one perform?

(b) Adam's clasps are often used to keep an appliance in place; what are the advantages of the design of this component?

(c) What other designs of such components are used to keep an appliance in place?

(d) Appliances may be designed with bite planes: when would you use an anterior bite plane and when would you use a posterior bite plane?

(e) What are the advantages of removable appliances?

Answer 1.3

(a)

- Active component — this is the site of delivery of the force to move a tooth/teeth

- Retentive component — this is the component that keeps the appliance in the mouth

- Anchorage component — provides resistance to unwanted teeth/tooth movement (every action has an equal and opposite reaction and hence there is always a reaction from the active components, and anchorage is the source of resistance to this movement)

- Baseplate — this holds all the components together

(b) Adam's clasp:
- Provides retention and anchorage

- Easy to adjust: anterior and posterior teeth

- Versatile: auxiliary fittings include double clasps, hooks for elastics, tubes for headgear attachment

(c)

- Ball hooks

- Southend clasp on the incisors

- Fitted labial bow

(d) The idea of an anterior bite plane is to open the bite to allow the posterior teeth to erupt while preventing the anterior teeth from erupting any more. As the posterior teeth erupt there is vertical development of the alveolus and the condyles will also grow. These are only used in a patient who is still actively growing. A posterior bite plane is almost the reverse where the anterior teeth are allowed to erupt while the posterior teeth are prevented from further eruption by the bite plane. This will cause a reduced overbite to increase, but again can only be used in a patient who is still actively growing.

(e) Advantages of removable appliances:
- Effective for simple tipping of favourably inclined teeth, (often mesial) over short distances
- Can transmit forces to blocks of teeth
- Easy to clean for patients
- Cheap to make and cheap clinically as use of minimal chair-side time
- Aesthetic
- Provide valuable anchorage
- Self-limiting

1.4 Fill in the missing details about tooth formation in the table below.

Tooth	Mineralisation commences	Eruption	Root formation completed
	Birth	6–7 years	9–10 years
Upper As			
Upper 3s			
Lower 5s			
Upper Ds			
Lower 8s			

Answer 1.4

Tooth	Mineralisation commences	Eruption	Root formation completed
Upper and lower 6s	Birth	6–7 years	9–10 years
Upper As	3–4 months in utero	7 months	1.5–2 years
Upper 3s	4–5 months	11–12 years	13–15 years
Lower 5s	2.25–2.5 years	11–12 years	13–14 years
Upper Ds	5 months in utero	12–16 months	2–2.5 years
Lower 8s	8–10 years	17–21 years	18–25 years

1.5 (a) Name two conditions that may result in delayed eruption of primary teeth.

(b) Name two local conditions and a systemic condition that may delay permanent tooth eruption (different from your answer to question 1.5 (a) above).

(c) How common is hypodontia in the primary and permanent dentition?

(d) Which gender is it most common in?

Answer 1.5

(a) Any two of the following conditions:
- Preterm birth
- Chromosomal abnormalities, eg Down syndrome, Turner syndrome
- Nutritional deficiency
- Hereditary gingival fibromatosis

(b) Local conditions — any two of the following:
- Supernumerary teeth
- Crowding
- Cystic change around the tooth follicle
- Ectopic position of the tooth germ

General conditions — any one of the following:
- Cleidocranial dysostosis
- Chromosomal abnormalities (Down syndrome, Turner syndrome)
- Nutritional deficiency
- Hereditary gingival fibromatosis
- Hypothyroidism
- Hypopituitarism

(c) The prevalence of hypodontia in the primary dentition is less than 1% and in the permanent dentition it is about 3.5–6.5% (Di Biase DD. *Dent Pract Dent Rec* 1971; **22**(3):95–108.)

(d) It is more common in females.

1.6 (a) What do you understand by the term 'infraocclusion' and how is it graded?

(b) An 11-year-old boy presents with an infraoccluded lower second deciduous molar. What percentage of primary molars are affected by this condition?

- 3–5%

- 5–8%

- 8–14%

- 15–20%

(c) How would you manage this problem?

(d) When would you refer for surgical removal?

(e) If there is a permanent successor and the second deciduous molar is still infraoccluded and is below the gingival tissue, what could have happened to the second deciduous molar? What will you need to consider after removal of the second deciduous molar?

Answer 1.6

(a) Infraoccluded teeth are teeth that fail to maintain their occlusal relationship with opposing or adjacent teeth. They were previously called submerged or ankylosed teeth. Infraocclusion most commonly affects the deciduous mandibular molars. It is graded as follows:

- Grade 1 — the occlusal surface of the tooth is above the contact point of the adjacent tooth.

- Grade II — the occlusal surface of the tooth is at the contact point of the adjacent tooth.

- Grade III — the occlusal surface of the tooth is below the contact point of the adjacent tooth.

(b) 8–14%

(c) Take a radiograph to see if there is a permanent successor. If there is one, it is likely that the infraoccluded second deciduous molar will exfoliate at the same time as the contralateral tooth, when the permanent successor starts to erupt.

(d) When there is no permanent successor and the tooth will probably 'disappear' below the gingival margin.

(e) The second deciduous molar may have ankylosed. Space maintenance will need to be considered after the extraction to allow eruption of the permanent molar.

1.7   A fit and healthy 12-year-old girl attends with her mother following an accident in which she fell off the apparatus at her gym club. She has banged both her upper anterior teeth. Examination reveals no extraoral injuries, but both the upper central incisors are mobile and the crowns are palatally displaced.

(a) What special tests would you carry out and why?

(b) The upper central incisors are fractured in the mid-third of the roots. What treatment would you carry out and how long must that treatment be done for?

(c) If the coronal portion of the tooth became non-vital what treatment would you carry out?

(d) If there were no root fractures, would your management have changed?

(e) If a dentoalveolar fracture had been diagnosed, would your management have changed and if so how?

Answer 1.7

(a) The following tests are recommended:
- Vitality tests of all upper and lower incisors as they may have been injured in the accident
- Periapical radiographs or an upper standard occlusal view to see if the roots are fractured

(b) Splint the teeth using a flexible splint that allows physiological tooth movement. A wire splint that is bonded to the injured teeth and one healthy tooth on either side of the injured teeth using acid-etched composite is easy to construct and well tolerated.

    The splint must be kept in place for 4 weeks. Previous treatment regimens used rigid splints for 2–3 months; this is now thought not to give the best results.

(c) The pulp should be extirpated up to the fracture line. The root canal is filled with non-setting calcium hydroxide to encourage barrier formation coronal to the fracture line. The calcium hydroxide should be changed every 3 months until the barrier forms, at which point the coronal root canal should be filled with gutta percha, and the tooth kept under review.

(d) The teeth are mobile and palatally displaced so they must have undergone some type of displacement injury. These would still require flexible splinting, usually for 2–3 weeks.

(e) Alveolar injuries require repositioning of tooth and splint for 4 weeks. Please see www.dentraumaguide.org for further info.

1.8   (a) What do you understand by the term 'behaviour management?'

(b) Name three types of communicative management.

(c) If a child is unable to tolerate dental treatment, drugs may be administered to help the child cope with the procedure. One way of drug delivery is inhalational sedation. What drug is commonly used with this method?

(d) Give two contraindications to the use of this drug.

(e) Name another sedative drug that may be used and the possible routes of delivery.

Answer 1.8

(a) Behaviour management is a way of encouraging a child to have a positive attitude towards oral health and healthcare so that treatment can be carried out. It is based on establishing communication while alleviating anxiety and fear, as well as building a trusting relationship between the dentist/therapist and delivering dental care.

(b) Any three of the following:
- Non-verbal communication
- Tell, show, do
- Voice control
- Distraction
- Positive reinforcement

(c) Nitrous oxide

(d) Any two of the following:
- Sickle cell disease
- Severe emotional disturbances
- Chronic obstructive pulmonary disease
- Cooperative patient

Drug-related dependency and first trimester pregnancy are also contraindications to the use of nitrous oxide. Sickle cell disease is a relative contraindication to the use of inhalational sedation; it is, however, the preferred alternative to general anaesthesia.

(e) Midazolam — oral, intranasal sedation

1.9   (a)   A fit and healthy 15-year-old girl complains of a wobbly upper tooth. Examination reveals that the tooth is a deciduous upper left canine and the permanent canine is not visible. Describe how you would determine whether there is an unerupted permanent canine.

(b)   You have a panoramic radiograph and a periapical view. Describe how you could use these images to determine the exact position of an unerupted tooth.

(c)   Name two other combinations of radiographs that could be used to localise the tooth.

(d)   What other imaging technique could be used to determine whether the tooth is buccally or palatally placed?

Answer 1.9

(a) Clinical examination — the angulation of lateral incisors may give a clue. A buccally placed canine tooth may push the apex of a lateral incisor palatally leaving the lateral incisor proclined. Palpation of the buccal sulcus and palate may reveal a bulge, which could be due to an underlying tooth. Radiographs are the definitive method of determining presence or absence of the permanent canine tooth.

(b) By using the parallax technique. When two views are taken with different angulations, any object that is further away from the tube will move in the same direction as the tube. This can be carried out in either the vertical or horizontal plane. With these two radiographs the tube has shifted from a near horizontal position in the panoramic radiograph to a much higher angulation in the periapical. If the canine tooth appears lower on the panoramic radiograph than it does on the periapical view then it has moved with the tube and is palatally situated and vice versa. If the tooth does not move at all then it is in the line of the arch.

(c) Any two of the following:
   • Two periapicals taken at different horizontal angulations

   • A periapical radiograph and an upper occlusal radiograph

   • An upper occlusal radiograph and a panoramic radiograph

(d) Cone-beam CT scan

1.10 What are the treatment options for impacted permanent canines when the deciduous predecessor has been lost? Give an advantage and disadvantage of each option.

Answer 1.10

Treatment option	Advantage	Disadvantage
No intervention and monitor impacted canine tooth	Easy	Still no tooth in gap — need prosthesis
Removal of impacted tooth	No possibility of cystic change	Surgical procedure; damage to adjacent teeth/structures; no tooth in gap — need prosthesis
Surgical exposure with orthodontically assisted eruption	Tooth ends up in proper position with an intact periodontal ligament	Surgery; patient needs to wear an orthodontic appliance (usually fixed appliance); prolonged treatment; tooth may not erupt
Transplantation of canine	Quick, tooth immediately put in place	Surgery; tooth may become ankylosed; loss of vitality; long-term prognosis not as good as teeth that erupt normally

1.11 (a) What types of appliance are the Andresen appliance, Frankel appliance and twin block appliance? How do they work?

(b) What age group of patients are they most effective in?

(c) Which type of malocclusion is most successfully treated with these appliances? What skeletal effects are thought to occur?

(d) Name two skeletal and two dental changes that are reported to occur with the use of these appliances.

Answer 1.11

(a) They are all functional appliances. A functional appliance is an orthodontic appliance that uses, guides or eliminates the forces generated by the orofacial musculature, tooth eruption and facial growth to correct a malocclusion.

(b) Growing children, preferably before the pubertal growth spurt as they use the forces of growth to correct the malocclusion.

(c) Their main use is to treat class II malocclusions, especially class II div I. However, they can also be used to treat anterior open bites and class III malocclusions.

There is still confusion about the exact effects of functional appliances but it is thought that they provide a combination of both skeletal and dental effects. With respect to the mandible, it is has been said that the mandible is stimulated to grow and the glenoid fossa remodels forwards as the appliances pull the condylar cartilage forwards, beyond the glenoid fossa. It is also claimed that forward maxillary growth is inhibited.

(d) Skeletal changes — any two of the following:
- Restraint or redirection of forward maxillary growth
- Optimisation of mandibular growth
- Forward movement of glenoid fossa
- Increase of lower facial height

Dental changes — any two of the following:
- Palatal tipping of upper incisors
- Labial tipping of lower incisors
- Inhibition of forward movement of maxillary molars
- Mesial and vertical eruption of mandibular molars

1.12 (a) What determine(s) the response of a tooth when force is applied to it?

(b) What changes are seen in the periodontal ligament when orthodontic forces are applied to teeth?

(c) Give five complications of orthodontic treatment.

(d) What force is usually used for orthodontic movement?

Answer 1.12

(a) The magnitude and duration of the force.

(b) Depending on the side:
- Tension side — stretching of the periodontal ligament fibres and stimulation of the osteoblasts on the bone surface, leading to bone deposition

- Compression side — compression of blood vessels, osteoclast accumulation which result in resorption of bone and formation of Howship lacunae into which fibrous tissue is deposited

(c) Any five of the following:
- Root resorption

- Enamel decalcification

- Gingivitis

- Trauma/ulceration from attachment

- Allergy from attachments, etc. (nickel)

- Relapse

- Incomplete treatment

- Loss of tooth vitality

- Patient dissatisfaction

(d) Typical forces used for orthodontic movement depend on the nature of the tooth movement required:
- Tipping: 50—75 g

- Translational: 100—150 g

- Rotational: 50—100 g

- Extrusion: 50 g

- Intrusion: 15—25 g

1.13 (a) In the current economic situation health providers need to show that orthodontic services are appropriately allocated. Name a commonly used index that categorises the urgency and need for orthodontic treatment.

(b) How many components are there in the index and what grades does this index incorporate?

Answer 1.13

(a) The index of orthodontic treatment need (IOTN). This was developed to help determine the likely impact of a malocclusion on an individual's dental health and psychological well-being.

(b) The IOTN has two components: the dental health and the aesthetic components. The dental health component has five grades and looks at traits that may affect the function and longevity of the dentition with grade 1 indicating no treatment need and grade 5 very great need.

The aesthetic component attempts to assess the aesthetic handicap of the malocclusion and the possible psychological effect and as such is difficult to grade. This part of the index consists of 10 photographs scored 1–10 where score 1 is the most aesthetically pleasing and 10 the least.

With regard to treatment need:

- Score 1–2: no treatment

- Score 3–4: slight need

- Score 5–7: moderate/borderline need

- Score 8–10: definite treatment need

The average score of the two components may be used, or as is more commonly done, the dental health component is assessed first; if this is graded 4–5 then it is not essential to assess the aesthetic component. If the dental health component is graded 3 then the aesthetic score is taken into account. An aesthetic score of 6 or above indicates a need for treatment.

1.14 (a) A 12-year-old girl complains of a 'gap between her upper central incisors' that she is getting teased about at school. Name four causes of a midline diastema.

(b) How would you determine the cause of the diastema?

(c) Once the potential cause of the diastema has been identified how should the patient be managed?

Answer 1.14

(a) Any four of the following:
- Physiological (central incisors erupt first and a diastema may be present until the upper canines erupt)
- Small teeth in large jaw (including peg laterals)
- Missing teeth
- Midline supernumerary, odontome
- Proclination of upper labial segment
- Prominent frenum (actual role is unclear although it is often cited as a cause)

(b) History and examination. In particular, look for:
- A prominent frenum. Pull the lip to put the frenum under tension and look for blanching of the incisive papilla
- Proclination of upper incisors
- Size of the teeth in the upper labial segment

Radiographs will help confirm if any teeth are missing or the presence of supernumerary teeth. A notch of the interdental bone between the upper central incisors is another sign of a prominent frenum.

(c) Consider the following management options:
- If the upper canines are unerupted and the diastema is < 3 mm then reassess after eruption of the canines.
- If the upper canines are unerupted and the diastema is > 3 mm orthodontic treatment may be needed when the canines erupt to approximate the incisors.
- If the upper canines are erupted then the incisors will require orthodontic approximation or restorative treatment to reduce the gap.
- If there is a prominent frenum, the patient should be referred for an opinion/treatment of the frenum. Surgical treatment would involve a frenectomy.
- If a supernumerary or odontome is present then refer for surgical removal.

- If teeth are missing, consider closing the midline diastema and a restorative option for the space created further laterally.

- If the upper labial segment is proclined, a full orthodontic assessment is needed to determine if it is treatable by orthodontics alone or may require surgical intervention at a later date.

- If the upper central and lateral incisors are very narrow with spacing then it may be possible to refer for restorative treatment to restore the teeth with composite, porcelain veneers or crowns to increase the width and minimise the gaps.

1.15 (a) How common is cleft lip and palate in western Europe?

- 1:200 births

- 1:700 births

- 1:1000 births

(b) At what age do most units carry out closure of the cleft lip?

- Neonatal period

- 3 months

- 6 months

- 9 months

(c) At what age do most units carry out repair of the cleft palate?

(d) Name two dental anomalies that often occur in cleft patients.

(e) At what stage may orthodontic treatment be needed?

(f) What may need to be carried out to aid eruption of the maxillary canine on the cleft side and when would this be done?

Answer 1.15

(a) 1:700 births

(b) 3 months

(c) Between 9 and 18 months

(d) Any two of the following:
  - Hypodontia

  - Supernumerary teeth

  - Delayed eruption of teeth

  - Hypoplasia

(e) In the mixed and/or permanent dentition:
  - Mixed dentition — proclination of upper incisors may be necessary if they erupt in lingual occlusion, otherwise orthodontic treatment is better deferred until just prior to alveolar bone grafting. Orthodontic expansion of the collapsed arch and alignment of upper incisors is required prior to alveolar bone grafting.

  - Permanent dentition — fixed appliances are usually required for alignment and space closure. Orthognathic surgery and associated orthodontic treatment is carried out when growth is completed. Patients classically have a hypoplastic maxilla with a class III malocclusion, and orthognathic surgery is considered for improvement in aesthetics and function.

(f) Alveolar bone grafting (grafting or placement of cancellous and/or cortical bone from another site, eg hip or tibia, to the cleft alveolus):
  - It is carried out to make a one-piece maxilla.

  - The grafting is usually done between the ages of 8 and 11 years, when the canine root is two-thirds formed.

  - It provides bone for the the canine to erupt into.

  - It provides bone as support for the alar base of the nose.

  - It provides an intact arch to allow tooth orthodontic movement.

  - It aids closure of any oronasal fistula.

1.16 (a) How would you advise parents to administer an appropriate fluoride dosage regimen at home for children in the following age groups:

- Up to 3 years

- 3—6 years

- From 7 years and young adults

- From 7 years and young adults (high caries risk/undergoing orthodontic treatment, those with special needs)

(b) What is the recommended professional intervention regarding fluoride for children in the following age groups?

- 3—6 years

- From 7 years and young adults

(c) Teeth start forming before the age of 6 months so why are fluoride supplements not given to younger children?

Answer 1.16

(a) Children aged up to 3 years:
- Parents should brush or supervise toothbrushing
- Use only a smear of toothpaste containing no less than 1000 ppm fluoride
- As soon as teeth erupt in the mouth, brush them twice daily

Children aged 3—6 years:
- Use a pea-sized amount of toothpaste containing 1350—1500 ppm fluoride
- Spit out after brushing and do not rinse (all children age 3—6 years)

Children aged from 7 years and young adults:
- Use fluoridated toothpaste (1350 ppm fluoride or above)
- Spit out after brushing and do not rinse

Children aged from 7 years and young adults (high caries risk/undergoing orthodontic treatment, those with special needs):
- Use fluoridated toothpaste (1350 ppm fluoride or above)
- Spit out after brushing and do not rinse
- Use fluoride mouthrinse daily (0.05% NaF) at a different time from brushing

(b) Children are placed into risk groups for caries

Children aged 3—6 years:
- Apply fluoride varnish to teeth twice yearly (2.2% F⁻)

Children aged 3—6 years (high risk)
- Apply fluoride varnish to teeth 2—3 times yearly (2.2% F⁻)
- Give advice about maximising benefit
- Reduce recall interval
- Investigate diet and assist to adopt good dietary practice
- Ensure medication is sugar-free or given to minimise cariogenic effect

Children aged from 7 years and young adults:
- Apply fluoride varnish to teeth twice yearly (2.2% F⁻)

Children aged from 7 years and young adults (high risk):
- Apply fluoride varnish to teeth 2–3 times yearly (2.2% F⁻)
- For those 8+ years with active caries prescribe daily fluoride rinse
- For those 10+ years with active caries prescribe 2800 ppm toothpaste
- For those 16+ years with active disease consider prescription of 5000 ppm toothpaste

In addition also consider the need to:
- Fissure seal permanent molars with resin sealant
- Investigate diet and assist adoption of good dietary practice

(c) Infants < 6 months of age do not have adequate renal function to excrete fluoride. Hence fluoride is contraindicated until children are at least 6 months old.

For more information see Department of Health. *Delivering Better Oral Health: An evidence-based toolkit for prevention*. London: DH, 2014.

1.17 (a) What are the factors that would put a child at high risk for developing caries?

(b) How would you carry out a diet analysis for a child?

(c) List four pieces of dietary advice that you would give to a parent/patient (child).

Answer 1.17

(a) Social factors:
- Family belonging to a lower socioeconomic group
- Irregular dental attendance
- Poor knowledge of dental disease
- Siblings with high caries rates

Dietary factors:
- Easily available sugary snacks
- Frequent sugar intake

Oral hygiene factors:
- Poor plaque control
- No fluoride

Medical history factors:
- Reduced salivary flow, or reduced buffering capacity
- Medically compromised
- Physical disability
- Cariogenic medicine taken long term
- High *Streptococcus mutans* and lactobacilli counts

(b) You need to ask the parents (carer) to record on a sheet the time, the food and the amount of everything that is eaten over a 3- to 4-day period. Try to include one day from the weekend as dietary habits are often different then.

(c) (Note: The term 'child' is routinely used for children over the age of 1.)
Encourage:
- Safe snacks (but beware of high-salt foods), eg nuts, fruit, bread, cheese
- Safe drinks — water, milk, tea with no sugar
- Tooth brushing

Limit:
- The frequency of sugar-containing food and drinks

- Sweets to mealtimes or one day a week

Avoid:
- Chewy sweets in particular

- Sweetened drinks in a bottle

Discourage:
- There is some controversy surrounding long-term breast-feeding, but breast milk has a higher lactose content compared with cows' milk. On-demand breast-feeding may give rise to caries, so try to discourage it.

Note: always try to be positive and do not make the parent feel guilty.

1.18 (a) What is meant by the terms balancing and compensating extractions?

(b) What is the likely effect of premature loss of a deciduous canine?

(c) Is the effect greater or less with the premature loss of a deciduous first molar than with a canine?

(d) What would you recommend in a crowded mouth requiring the unilateral loss of an upper canine?

(e) What is the effect of premature loss of deciduous second molars?

(f) Do you compensate or balance the premature loss of deciduous second molars?

Answer 1.18

(a) A balancing extraction is the extraction of the same or adjacent tooth on the opposite side of the same arch. A compensating extraction is the extraction of same or adjacent tooth in the opposing arch on the same side.

(b) The primary effect of early loss of deciduous teeth in a crowded mouth is localised crowding. The extent will depend on several factors, including the patient's age, extent of existing crowding and the site of the early tooth loss. In crowding, adjacent teeth will move into the extraction space, hence a centreline shift will occur with the unilateral loss of a deciduous canine.

(c) A centreline shift will occur to a lesser degree with the unilateral loss of a deciduous first molar compared with a deciduous canine.

(d) The unilateral loss of a canine should be balanced as the correction of a centreline discrepancy is likely to need a fixed appliance and prevention is preferable to dealing with the problem.

(e) The premature loss of deciduous second molars is associated with forward migration of the first permanent molars. This is greater if the deciduous second molars are lost before eruption of the first permanent molars, so if possible, delay extraction of deciduous second molars until the first permanent molars are in occlusion.

(f) Neither

1.19 (a) An anterior open bite can occur with which types of malocclusion?

(b) Give a simple classification of the causes of an anterior open bite.

(c) An anterior open bite caused by one factor is relatively straightforward to treat. Which factor is this?

(d) What other occlusal features may you see in this situation?

(e) How will you treat an open bite due to the factor in (c)?

Answer 1.19

(a) It can occur in a class I, class II or class III malocclusion.

(b) Skeletal causes:
- Increase in lower anterior face height (increased lower face height or increased maxillary to mandibular plane angle)
- Localized failure of alveolar growth

Soft tissue causes:
- Endogenous tongue thrust

Habits:
- Digit sucking

(c) Digit sucking

(d) Occlusal features that may be seen in this situation:
- Retroclined lower incisors
- Proclined upper incisors
- Unilateral buccal segment crossbite with mandibular displacement

(e) It is best not to make a big fuss of digit sucking. Most children grow out of the habit and the malocclusion usually corrects itself after several years. However, if there are other aspects of the malocclusion that need treatment, this should not be delayed. Various appliances may help to break the habit.

1.20 (a) Name five ways in which fluoride is administered to children.

(b) Give an advantage and disadvantage of each of the methods you have listed.

Method	Advantage	Disadvantage

Answer 1.20

(a) Any five of the methods listed in the table in answer (b) can be given here.

(b)

Method	Advantage	Disadvantage
General water supply	Very cheap, available to everyone, does not rely on patient compliance	Not readily available in the UK as there is opposition to fluoridation; varies with where the child lives
Milk, eg school milk schemes	Cheap; not carrying out extra regimen	Not available to all children
Salt	Cheap, not carrying out an extra regimen	Not in the UK
Toothpaste	Daily delivery; not an extra drug as patient already using toothpaste	Relies on patient brushing teeth
Gel	High fluoride content	Relies on dental professional; care required not to ingest gel
Varnishes	High fluoride content; may result in arrest of early lesions; can use them to introduce children to dental care	Relies on dental professional; care required not to ingest varnish
Rinses	Can use as part of oral hygiene regimen	Not good for young children
Tablets	Topical and systemic effects; have to take a tablet	Relies on patient/parent compliance

1.21   A fit and healthy 6-year-old girl attends your practice with her mother complaining of intermittent pain from the mandibular, right second primary molar (LRE). The pain is set off by cold drinks, it does not disturb her sleep and has not required pain relief (analgesics).

(a) What is your diagnosis?

(b) What are your treatment options because the child's mother is keen to save the tooth?

(c) What different medications could you use?

(d) What would be your definitive restoration of choice?

(e) What are the signs of irreversible pulpitis and what would be your treatment options for a tooth that exhibited them?

Answer 1.21

(a) Reversible pulpitis: provoked pain of short duration relieved with over-the-counter analgesics, by brushing or on the removal of the stimulus.

(b) Teeth exhibiting signs/symptoms of reversible pulpitis are candidates for pulpotomy or indirect pulp therapy (IPT):

- IPT arrests the carious process and provides conditions conducive to the formation of reactionary dentine beneath the stained dentine, with remineralisation of remaining carious dentine; this promotes pulpal healing and preserves/maintains the vitality of the pulp tissue.

- Pulpotomy: involves removal of the coronally inflamed pulp and maintenance of the radicular pulp, which is reversibly inflamed or healthy.

(c)

- IPT: hard-setting calcium hydroxide or reinforced glass ionomer cement

- Pulpotomy: 15.5% ferric sulphate solution, mineral trioxide aggregate (MTA), calcium hydroxide

(d) Preformed metal crown (PMC) to achieve optimum external coronal seal

(e)

- Pulpectomy or extraction

- Irreversible pulpitis: a history of spontaneous unprovoked toothache, a sinus tract, excessive mobility not associated with trauma or exfoliation, furcation/apical radiolucency or radiographic evidence of internal/external resorption

1.22 (a) Select the most appropriate word to fill the blanks in this paragraph about development of the maxilla and mandible.

The maxilla is derived from the .... pharyngeal arch and undergoes .... ossification. Maxillary growth ceases .... in girls than in boys. The mandible is derived from the .... pharyngeal arch and is a membranous bone. The mandible elongates with growth at the condylar cartilage, at the same time bone is laid down at the .... vertical ramus and resorbed on the .... margin. Mandibular growth ceases .... than maxillary growth and is .... in girls than in boys.

   1 first, second, third

   2 intramembranous, endochondral

   3 earlier, later

   4 anterior, posterior

   (b) What is the difference between endochondral and intramembranous ossification? Give an example of where each occurs in the head.

Answer 1.22

(a) The maxilla is derived from the *first* pharyngeal arch and undergoes *intramembranous* ossification. Maxillary growth ceases *earlier* in girls (15 years and 17 years in boys). The mandible is derived from the *first* pharyngeal arch and is a membranous bone. The mandible elongates with growth at the condylar cartilage, at the same time bone is laid down at the *posterior* vertical ramus and resorbed on the *anterior* margin. Mandibular growth ceases *later* than maxillary growth and is *earlier* in girls (average 17 years in girls and 19 years in boys).

(b) Endochondral ossification occurs at cartilaginous growth centres where chondroblasts lay down a matrix of cartilage within which ossification occurs. This occurs at the synchondroses of the cranial base. Intramembranous ossification is the process in which bone is both laid down within fibrous tissue; there is no cartilaginous precursor. This occurs in the bones of the vault of the skull and the face.

1.23 (a) List two localised and three generalised causes of abnormalities in the structure of enamel.

(b) What do you understand by the term enamel hypoplasia and how does it differ from hypocalcification?

(c) Name three disturbances of dentine formation.

(d) What do you understand by the term Turner teeth?

Answer 1.23

(a) Localised causes — any two of the following:
  - Infection
  - Trauma
  - Irradiation

Generalised causes — any two of the following:
  - Amelogenesis imperfecta
  - Infections: prenatal (rubella, syphilis); postnatal (measles)
  - At birth: premature birth; prolonged labour
  - Fluoride
  - Nutritional deficiencies
  - Down syndrome
  - Idiopathic

(b) Hypoplasia is a disturbance in the formation of the matrix of enamel which gives rise to pitted and grooved enamel. Hypocalcification is a disturbance in mineralisation (calcification) of the enamel and gives rise to opaque white enamel.

(c) Any two of the following:
  - Dentinogenesis imperfecta
  - Dentinal dysplasia type I and II
  - Fibrous dysplasia of dentine
  - Regional odontodysplasia
  - Ehlers—Danlos syndrome
  - Vitamin D resistant rickets
  - Vitamin D dependent rickets
  - Hypophosphatasia

(d) This is caused by infection from a deciduous tooth affecting the developing underlying permanent tooth. It results in abnormal enamel and dentine.

2
Restorative Dentistry

2.1   (a) What chemicals are currently used to bleach teeth? What is the
mode of action for each of them?

(b) What are the side effects/complications of vital bleaching and when
would bleaching not be indicated?

(c) Microabrasion can be used to alter the colour of teeth. What is it
and for what types of discoloration would it be indicated?

Answer 2.1

(a) Hydrogen peroxide and carbamide peroxide are the commonly used chemicals for tooth bleaching.

Carbamide peroxide is broken down into hydrogen peroxide and urea, so in both cases the bleaching is actually done by hydrogen peroxide. This is a very small molecule, which penetrates enamel and dentine, and dissociates into a superoxide ion and water. The superoxide ion is thought to bleach teeth by oxidising the pigments that are trapped in the stains.

(b)
- Sensitivity of vital teeth often occurring after bleaching, which may necessitate the use of fluoride mouthwash or some other type of dentine desensitiser
- The bleaching possibly fading over time and needing to be redone
- Possibility of resorption of teeth, especially in those techniques that use heat to activate the hydrogen peroxide
- Soft-tissue chemical burns
- Potential adverse effects on restorative materials

Vital bleaching would not be indicated in the following situations:
- Patients who have severe widespread discolouration of their teeth, such as tetracycline staining or pitting hypoplasia
- Adolescent patients with large pulp chambers
- Teeth with large or defective restorations
- Teeth with apical pathology
- Teeth that are fractured or excessively worn
- Teeth with deep surface cracks
- Pregnant women
- Patients with unrealistic expectations
- Teeth that are already sensitive to thermal changes

(c) Microabrasion is a technique in which no more than the outer 100 μm of enamel is removed by using a combination of abrasion and erosion. Hydrochloric acid is used in a slurry on the tooth, applied with a rubber cup over the enamel surface.

Indications: used mainly for isolated discoloured spots rather than generalised discoloration, in particular fluorosis, brown mottling and idiopathic stains, before veneer placement.

2.2 (a) It is now considered normal practice to prepare teeth to receive a porcelain veneer restoration. What are the advantages of tooth preparation before veneer placement?

(b) In what situations would a veneer not be indicated?

(c) What are the stages involved in luting a veneer?

Answer 2.2

(a)

- The bond strength is greater when the tooth is prepared.

- The emergence profile of the restoration is better and results in better gingival health.

- The tooth is not increased in size, which gives a better aesthetic outcome.

(b)

- If the tooth was subject to abnormally heavy occlusion, eg in the case of a patient with bruxism

- Where the margins of the restoration would have to be placed way below the gingival margin

- If the tooth had already received large restorations, in which case it may be more sensible to opt for a full coverage restoration rather than a veneer

- Where there was inadequate remaining tooth structure for bonding or where it remained of poor quality

- Poor oral hygiene

(c)

- The tooth to receive the veneer should be isolated and then cleaned with pumice. Care must be taken to ensure that there is no oil contaminating the pumice because this will affect the bond.

- The veneer should not be tried on the model because stone will contaminate the fit surface of the veneer.

- Apply the appropriate silane coupling agent to the fit surface of the veneer and let it dry.

- Try the veneer on the tooth with a drop of water or in paste on the fit surface. This helps in terms of shade assessment.

- Carry out any adjustment of the fit and proximal contacts.

- Remove and try in paste with ethyl alcohol and, if need be, re-etch the fit surface of the veneer with 37% orthophosphoric acid.

- Reapply silane coupling agent

- Etch tooth and apply dentine-bonding agent

- Place unfilled resin on tooth and veneer

- Apply filled resin lute to veneer and gently seat the veneer; avoid excess pressure

- Spot cure the incisal edge

- Remove excess resin lute and floss the contacts

- Cure completely

- Carry out minimal finishing with a bur because this is best left until the resin has set, which is usually 24 h later. When fully set a diamond finishing bur can be used along with finishing strips and discs.

2.3 (a) What changes may occur to the tooth structure as a result of endodontic treatment?

   (b) What are your options for restoration in an endodontic treated tooth?

Answer 2.3

(a) Endodontic treatment is said to 'weaken' the remaining tooth structure. A number of factors have been implicated:

- The preparation of the access cavity, leading to changes in architecture, especially the lost of marginal ridge and occlusal isthmus

- Changes in property of the dentine: collagen depletion with predisposition to fracture

- Changes in proprioception: non-vital teeth apparently have higher pain threshold

- The original insult, leading to need for endodontic treatment, eg caries, cracks, trauma

(b) Restoration of anterior and posterior teeth differs but the aim is to create a good coronal seal. Separate into temporary and definitive restoration:

Temporary:

- Zinc oxide/calcium sulphate, eg Cavit

- Intermediate restorative material (IRM): zinc oxide—eugenol base material

- Glass ionomer cement (GIC)

Permanent:

- Consider if post required

- Anterior teeth:

  - Direct composite restoration ± post

  - Crowns

- Posterior teeth:

  - Marginal ridges are intact — composite or amalgam if:

    - marginal ridge compromised

    - complex amalgams

    - composite with cuspal coverage

    - onlays/overlay in gold

    - indirect composite/porcelain

Full-coverage crown with ferrule for more predictable restoration. A ferrule is a band of crown material that completely encircles the tooth and is between the dentine—core interface and the cervical crown margin.

Nayyar cores are useful in posterior teeth because amalgam can be packed 2—3 mm into the canal orifice, avoiding the need for a post and providing an orifice seal.

2.4 (a) Drugs can be delivered locally into periodontal pockets. However, they should not be used without root surface instrumentation at the site. Why?

(b) In what circumstances would this method of drug delivery be appropriate?

(c) What advantages are there to using this method of drug delivery?

(d) Name two different types of delivery device for the local delivery of drugs into a periodontal pocket. What is the difference between them?

(e) Name two drugs commonly delivered by this route.

Answer 2.4

(a) Root surface instrumentation is needed because plaque and calculus in the pocket will decrease the ability of the drug to get into the tissues of the periodontal pocket

If deposits of plaque and calculus remain this will favour re-colonisation of the pocket by bacteria; the periodontal treatment and maintenance are therefore likely to be less effective or ineffective.

(b)
- As an adjunct to drainage and root surface debridement in the management of a periodontal abscess
- For areas of resistant disease
- In the management of furcation-involved teeth
- In the management of aggressive periodontitis

(c) High levels of the drug can be delivered directly to the area where they are needed, and can be maintained for a period of time in the gingival crevicular fluid. When drugs are given systemically, the concentrations rise and fall, whereas these spikes in concentration are not seen with local drug delivery systems.

There is also less likelihood of adverse effects from the drugs.

(d)
- Sustained-release device that will release a drug over 24 h
- Controlled-delivery device that will release a drug for over 24 h

(e)
- Chlorhexidine
- Tetracycline
- Minocycline
- Doxycycline
- Metronidazole
- Azithromycin

2.5 (a) Name the different categories of definitive tooth-coloured crowns that can be used.

(b) What are the advantages and disadvantages of having a metal substructure to a tooth-coloured crown?

(c) Name two commercially available dental materials from which all-ceramic restorations are made.

(d) Name two methods of constructing an all-ceramic monolithic crown.

(e) Name two differences between crowns constructed using these techniques.

Answer 2.5

(a)

- Metal—ceramic/porcelain fused to metal (PFM)/bonded crown
- All ceramic
- Composite (direct/indirect)

(b)

- The main advantages of metal—ceramic crowns over composite and all-ceramic crowns are:

  - Laboratory studies have shown metal—ceramic restorations to be stronger.

  - The ability to have metal lingual and occlusal surfaces makes these types of restorations more conservative of tooth tissue.

- The main disadvantages of metal—ceramic crowns over composite and all-ceramic crowns are:

  - Metal—ceramic restorations are not translucent and often have a metal collar, which may be noticeable at the cervical margin. Therefore they may have inferior aesthetics.

(c) Any two of the following:
- Leucite-reinforced glass ceramic

- Lithium disilicate-reinforced glass ceramic

- Feldspathic porcelain

- Alumina

- Zirconia

(d)

- CAD/CAM

CAD/CAM is an acronym for computer-aided design/computer-aided manufacturing.

Dental CAD/CAM technology is available for use in dental practices and dental laboratories. This enables dentists and laboratory technicians to design restorations on a computer screen. The CAD/CAM computer displays a three-dimensional customised image of the prepared tooth, or model of the prepared tooth, by digitally capturing the data with an optical scanner. The dentist or technician designs the final restoration from the data. Once the final restoration has been designed, the crown is milled from a single block of ceramic material. The shade is then adjusted in the colouring solution, and sintered in an oven.

- Pressed

Lost-wax hot-pressing technique

(e) The differences in the crowns are shown below.

CAD/CAM crowns (zirconia)	Pressed (lithium disilicate)
Zirconia based, eg Zirkon, Procero, Lava)	Glass based, eg Emax
Greater opacity	More translucent
Higher strength	Low strength
Strength not influenced by type of cement used (conventional* or resin cement). Zirconia cannot be etched	Must be etched and bonded with resin cement, which increases the strength

*For example, zinc phosphate.

2.6 (a) What compounds are used for bleaching teeth?

(b) How do bleaches work to remove discolouration from teeth?

(c) What are the potential side effects of bleaching a tooth?

(d) What non-vital bleaching techniques are there? Please describe the key features of each.

(e) What is the recommended concentration of bleaching agent used? List other specific recommendations.

Answer 2.6

(a)
- Carbamide peroxide
- Hydrogen peroxide
- Sodium perborate

(b) All bleaches form hydrogen peroxide, which is a powerful oxidising agent that breaks down into oxygen and free radicals. The molecules that discolour the teeth are broken down by the free radicals and oxygen and the resulting small molecules are lost from the tooth by diffusion.

(c)
- Sensitivity
- Shade regression
- Cervical resorption
- Irritation of the gingivae

(d) **Walking bleach technique**
- The gutta percha (GP) is removed from a satisfactorily root canal treated tooth to a level of 2—3 mm below the epithelial attachment.
- The cut face of the root canal GP is sealed with about 2—3 mm of glass ionomer cement. It is important to get the barrier at the correct level to ensure that the whole of the crown is bleached but to prevent material seeping through dentine below the epithelial attachment as cervical resorption could occur.
- The bleaching material is sealed in the cavity with a pledget of cotton wool and a temporary restoration placed. Some workers suggest etching the cavity to open up dentinal tubules prior to bleaching, although this is not universally accepted.
- The original technique used sodium perborate, although it is possible to use carbamide or hydrogen peroxide.
- The patient is reviewed after 2—3 days and the procedure repeated until the desired colour is achieved.

Inside-outside technique

- The first part of the technique is similar to the first two steps in the walking bleach technique.

- The access cavity is then left open.

- The patient applies bleaching solution into the access cavity and into a bleaching tray every 2 hours during the day time and also wears the bleaching tray overnight.

- The bleaching solution used is usually 10% carbamide peroxide.

- The advantages of this technique are that it allows the tooth to be bleached from both the internal and external aspects, but does require a very compliant and dextrous patient

In-surgery technique

- The tooth in question is isolated with rubber dam

- The access cavity is opened

- Hydrogen peroxide (up to 35%) is placed in the access cavity

- Activated with light or laser to speed up the activation of the free radicals

Individual tooth bleaching using trays

- Bleaching agent is applied to a single tooth by using a tray which only has a space for the agent to cover the discoloured tooth.

- This may be combined with the walking bleach technique in order to speed up the bleaching process.

(e)

- Between 0.1% and 6% hydrogen peroxide is the recommended concentration. Products containing or releasing between 0.1% and 6% hydrogen peroxide cannot be used on any person aged under 18 years except where such use is intended wholly for the purpose of treating or preventing disease.

- Tooth-whitening products containing or releasing between 0.1% and 6% hydrogen peroxide can be sold only to dental practitioners.

- For each cycle of use, the first use can be carried out only by dental practitioners, or under their direct supervision if an equivalent level of safety is ensured.

- The Cosmetic Products (Safety) (Amendment) Regulations 2012 (implementing Directive 2011/84 EU, which amends Directive 76/768/EEC) came into force on 31 October 2012.

2.7 (a) What is the difference between a craze, a crack and a fracture in a tooth?

(b) Describe the symptoms a patient may complain of if they have a cracked cusp/tooth.

(c) What is the mechanism that causes the pain?

(d) What special test could you use to aid diagnosis of a cracked cusp/tooth and what would the test show?

(e) How would you treat a tooth with a cracked cusp?

Answer 2.7

(a)

- A craze is an area of weakness in tooth structure where further propagation will result in a crack. They can be identified with fibre optic illumination.

- A crack is a definite break in the continuity of the tooth structure which begins in the enamel or the cementum, but no separation is evident. They can be seen with fibre-optic illumination, or in good clinical light.

- A fracture is when the tooth structure has separated into two or more distinct pieces and is visible clinically and often radiographically.

(b) The symptoms will depend on the health of the pulp. Initially it will be sharp pain, usually from a posterior tooth, which occurs on biting, but the patient may notice that it is worse when the bite is released (rebound pain). The pain is usually of short duration, and it may also be triggered by changes in temperature, eg cold. If it progresses to irreversible pulpitis the patient will have symptoms of irreversible pulpitis, ie, continuous throbbing pain that is worse on lying down. Often poorly localised and may radiate along the jaw.

(c) Movement of the cracked pieces of tooth cause movement of fluid in the dentinal tubules, which stimulates Aδ pain fibres.

(d)

- Clinical examination of a dry tooth with a good light from different angles, and if necessary using transillumination and magnification, will often show a crack.

- Place something (tooth sleuth, cotton wool, rubber dam, etc.) between each tooth and over individual cusps and get the patient to bite, which will cause the crack to open and elicit pain.

- The second test can also be carried out after placing methylene blue dye on the tooth, which will highlight the crack.

- Vitality tests show the tooth to be vital (provided the pulpitis is reversible).

- Radiographs often do not show up small cracks.

(e)

- If the tooth had symptoms of irreversible pulpitis, a root canal treatment would be indicated, or extraction if the patient declines root canal treatment.

- Removal of the restoration and further investigation of the size of the crack; if it is extending into the pulp, root canal treatment will be required.

- A temporary measure may be required to allow the pulp to settle and the tooth to be reassessed. This may involve placement of an adhesive restoration such as composite resin, glass ionomer or a bonded amalgam. As a very temporary measure an orthodontic band around the tooth, or a copper ring, may be placed around the tooth.

- Long-term restoration will involve a full-coverage crown or partial-coverage onlay or adhesive restoration to splint the remaining tooth structure.

2.8 (a) When preparing a root canal both files and reamers may be used. What is the difference between these two types of instrument?

(b) What requirements should be met prior to obturating a root canal?

(c) If there is evidence of serous fluid seeping into the canal what does this suggest?

(d) What features would an ideal root canal filling material have?

(e) Gutta percha (GP) is a commonly used root canal filling material. What techniques are available to obturate a root canal with this material?

(f) How would you assess whether a root canal filling that you have done has been successful?

Answer 2.8

(a) A file has much tighter spirals along its length and produces a cutting action when it is withdrawn from the root canal whereas a reamer has a looser spiral and is used by rotating and withdrawing.

(b) The root canal must be completely prepared and be dry and asymptomatic.

(c) It suggests inflammation of the periapical tissues is present.

(d)

- Non-irritant to periapical/periradicular tissues
- Easy to handle, insert into the root canal and remove if the root canal filling fails
- Radiopaque, but should not stain the tooth tissue, or be visible through the coronal tooth tissue
- Sterile
- Bacteriostatic
- Provide a good seal to the root canal and be stable and not shrink, and be impervious to water or liquids

(e)

- Lateral condensation — warm or cold
- Vertical condensation
- Thermo-mechanical condensation
- Thermo-plasticised GP
- Single point techniques
- Carrier-based techniques

(f)

- Patient history — absence of any reports of pain, swelling, discharge, mobility of the tooth
- Clinical examination — functional tooth, integrity of the restoration in/on the tooth, absence of swelling, mobility, a sinus, tenderness to percussion, tenderness to palpation

- Radiographic findings — good quality obturation to the appropriate length

- Depending on the time since obturation there may well still be a radiolucency that is present. However, if sufficient time has elapsed since the last appointment then shrinkage or disappearance of the radiolucency.

  up to 4 years?

2.9 (a) What is the difference between reattachment and new attachment?

   (b) What is meant by the term guided tissue regeneration (GTR) and why is it desirable in periodontal healing?

   (c) What factors would be considered desirable when designing a material for GTR?

   (d) Which of the following materials used in GTR are resorbable and which are non-resorbable?

Material	Resorbable/non-resorbable
Collagen	
Polylactic acid	
Teflon (ePTFE) (expanded poly-tetrafluoroethylene)	

Answer 2.9

(a) Reattachment means the reunion of the connective tissue to a root surface that had been separated by either incision or an injury whereas the term new attachment means the union of connective tissue with a root surface that was previously pathogenically altered.

(b) Following periodontal treatment it is hoped that a functional attachment with periodontal fibres embedded in bone at one end and cementum at the other will occur. However, the junctional epithelium has a large regenerative capacity and will grow down and cover exposed connective tissue creating a long epithelial attachment with the root if not excluded from the wound. Using a membrane it is possible to guide the tissue regeneration to prevent epithelial cells from gaining access to the root surface and also preventing gingival connective tissue from contacting the root surface. It also creates a small space to allow stem cells from the periodontal ligament and alveolar bone to migrate, differentiate and hopefully repopulate the exposed root surface to form a new attachment.

(c)

- Biocompatibility
- Ease of clinical use
- Impermeable to cells
- Able to maintain the space created
- Tissue integration

(d)

Material	Resorbable/Non-resorbable
Collagen	Resorbable
Polylactic acid	Resorbable
Teflon (ePTFE)	Non-resorbable

2.10 (a) What information can be determined from periodontal probing?

(b) What measurement gives the most accurate assessment with regards to periodontal destruction and why?

(c) How much pressure should be applied on the probe when carrying out periodontal probing?

(d) What factors may influence the results of periodontal probing?

(e) Where on a tooth should you assess pocket depths?

(f) How would you assess the furcation area of a tooth with a periodontal probe?

Answer 2.10

(a)

- Pocket depth, ie distance from the gingival margin to the base of the gingival pocket

- Presence of bleeding after probing

- Attachment loss, distance in millimetres from the cementoenamel junction (CEJ) to the base of the gingival pocket

(b) The measurement of attachment loss from the CEJ to the base of the pocket, as it gives a true idea of how much connective tissue attachment loss from the root surface there has been; also, it is not influenced by false pocketing.

(c) 0.25 N

(d)

- Pressure applied to the probe and the angle that is inserted

- Thickness of the probe

- The contour of the tooth

- The presence of calculus

- Inflammation of the gingival tissues

- Position of the gingival margin

- Patient tolerance

(e) It is normal practice to probe in six places — mesial, mid and distal on both the buccal and lingual aspects.

(f) Pass the probe horizontally between the roots to measure loss of periodontal support. Various classification systems are available, eg Hamp et al. (Hamp, SE, Nyman, S, Lindhe, J. *J Clin Periodontol* 1975; **2**(3):126−35):
- Degree 1 — loss of support less than one-third the buccolingual width of the tooth

- Degree 2 — loss of support less than one-third the buccolingual width of the tooth but not encompassing the total width of the furcation area

- Degree 3 — through-and-through defect

2.11 (a) What do you understand by the following terms?

- **Biological width**

- **Attached gingivae**

- **Free gingivae**

(b) What is the function of gingival crevicular fluid?

(c) Why might clinicians wish to sample it and what techniques are used to get such a sample?

Answer 2.11

(a) Biological width is the combined width of the attachment to the tooth from the most coronal aspect of the junctional epithelium to the most apical attachment of the gingival fibres at the level of the alveolar bone crest.

The oral gingivae are divided into attached and free gingivae. The free gingiva extends from the most coronal aspect of the gingival contour (free gingival margin) to the free gingival groove. Apical to the free gingiva is the attached gingiva, which extends from the free gingival groove to the mucogingival junction.

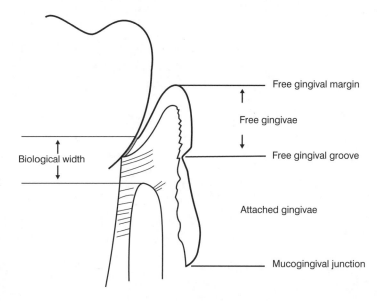

(b) It is an inflammatory exudate from the gingival crevicular tissues and forms part of the defence mechanism of the dento-gingival junction as it carries antimicrobial factors into the crevice. It is thought to wash debris such as dead epithelial cells and bacteria out of the crevice. It also carries polymorphonuclear leukocytes, macrophages, lysozyme and immunoglobulins into the crevice, which have an antimicrobial effect.

(c) There is a move to find diagnostic tests for periodontal disease activity, and it is possible that the crevicular fluid may contain components that could be used as reliable biomarkers. Tools used would be microcapillary tubes, absorbent paper and gingival washing.

2.12 (a) What is the difference between scaling and root surface debridement?

(b) Give a brief description of the following periodontal instruments and when you would choose to use them.

- **Scalers**

- **Curettes**

- **Hoes**

(c) What are the types of mechanised instruments used for periodontal treatment? Give a brief description of how they work.

Answer 2.12

(a) Scaling is the removal of deposits of plaque and calculus from a tooth surface whereas root surface debridement is the removal of subgingival deposits of plaque, calculus and necrotic cementum. It is no longer considered necessary to remove large amounts of cementum in order to leave the root surface smooth and hard, as this is detrimental to the tooth, but rather to disrupt the subgingival biofilm so that the environment is more likely to promote healing.

(b) The working end of a scaler in cross-section is an inverted triangle shape with two cutting edges superiorly and a blunt inferior edge. The tip of the scaler ends in a point. They tend to be used for removal of supragingival deposits or removing calculus that is located just below the gingival margin.

Curettes may be universal or site specific (Gracey curettes). The working part of the instrument has a spoon-shaped blade with two curved cutting edges if universal or a single cutting edge if site specific. A universal curette may be used throughout the whole mouth for removal of supra- and subgingival calculus. A whole set of site-specific curettes would be needed to access the whole mouth but they may be used for removal of supra- and subgingival calculus.

Hoes have one cutting edge bevelled at 45 degrees to the shank and which is designed in four different positions to create instruments that can be used on the mesial, distal, buccal and lingual surfaces of teeth. They can be used on all tooth surfaces but are particularly good for subgingival scaling and root surface debridement.

(c)
- Ultrasonic — converts electrical energy into high-frequency vibrations

- Magnetostrictive — in these the pattern of vibration of the tip is elliptical and so all sides of the tip are active

- Piezoelectric units — in these the pattern of vibration is back and forth so the two sides of the tip are active

- Sonic handpieces — uses air pressure to cause vibrations but vibrates at a slower rate than an ultrasonic instrument

- Air abrasive systems — these appear to be more useful in removing surface stains than removing deposits of calculus

2.13 (a) Name five causes of intrinsic discolouration of vital teeth.

(b) The appearance of discoloured teeth can be improved by methods which require tooth preparation and those that do not. Please name two of each.

(c) How would you remove extrinsic staining from tooth surfaces?

Answer 2.13

(a) Any five of the following:
- Trauma resulting in pulpal death
- Fluorosis
- Tetracycline staining
- Amelogenesis imperfecta
- Dentinogenesis imperfecta

(b) Methods requiring preparation:
- Veneer
- Crown

Methods not requiring preparation:
- Bleaching
- Microabrasion
- Composite veneers

(c) Removing extrinsic stains:
- Polishing the surfaces with pumice slurry and water or prophylaxis paste
- Ultrasonic cleaners
- Bleaching

2.14 (a) What do you understand by the terms primary dentine, secondary dentine and tertiary dentine?

(b) What is the difference between internal and external resorption?

(c) Are teeth with internal resorption likely to be vital or non-vital?

(d) Are teeth with external resorption likely to be vital or non-vital?

(e) Replacement resorption may result in ankylosis. What are the signs of ankylosis?

Answer 2.14

(a) Primary dentine is formed before eruption or within 2–3 years after eruption and consists of mainly of circumpulpal dentine. It also includes mantle dentine in the crown and the hyaline layer and granular layer in the root.

    Secondary dentine is the regular dentine that is formed during the life of the tooth and laid down in the floor and ceiling of the pulp chamber. It is a physiological type of dentine after the full length of root has formed.

    Tertiary dentine can be divided into reparative and reactionary dentine, both of which are laid down in response to noxious stimuli. Reactionary dentine is laid down in response to mild stimuli whereas reparative dentine is laid down directly beneath the path of injured dentinal tubules as a response to stronger stimuli and are irregular.

(b) Internal resorption starts within the pulp chamber of a tooth. External resorption starts on the surface of a tooth, most commonly on the root surface.

(c) Internal resorption can occur only in vital teeth (or partially vital teeth).

(d) External resorption may occur on vital or non-vital teeth.

(e) An ankylosed tooth:
- Has a different sound from a normal tooth when it is percussed, often described as a cracked china sound
- Lacks periodontal membrane space on a radiograph
- Has no physiological mobility
- May become infraoccluded as the jaw grows around it

2.15 Complete the table with regard to the basic periodontal examination (BPE) using the options given below.

Code	Finding on probing	Treatment
0		
1		Oral hygiene instruction (OHI)
2		
3	Probing depth 3.5–5.5 mm *(black band partially visible, indicating pocket of 4–5 mm)*	
4		
*	Furcation involvement	OHI, root surface debridement (RSD). Assess the need for more complex treatment; referral to a specialist may be indicated

Findings

- No pockets > 3.5 mm, no calculus/overhangs, no bleeding after probing *(black band completely visible)*

- Probing depth > 5.5 mm *(black band entirely within the pocket, indicating pocket of 6 mm)*

- No pockets > 3.5 mm, no calculus/overhangs, but bleeding after probing *(black band completely visible)*

- No pockets > 3.5 mm, but supra- or subgingival calculus/overhangs, possible bleeding on probing *(black band completely visible)*

Treatment

- OHI, RSD

- OHI, RSD. Assess the need for more complex treatment; referral to a specialist may be indicated

- No need for periodontal treatment

- OHI, removal of plaque retentive factors, including all supra- and subgingival calculus

Answer 2.15

Code	Finding on probing	Treatment
0	No pockets > 3.5 mm, no calculus/overhangs, no bleeding after probing *(black band completely visible)*	No need for periodontal treatment
1	No pockets > 3.5 mm, no calculus/overhangs, but bleeding after probing *(black band completely visible)*	OHI
2	No pockets > 3.5 mm, but supra- or subgingival calculus/overhangs, possible bleeding on probing *(black band completely visible)*	OHI, removal of plaque retentive factors, including all supra- and subgingival calculus
3	Probing depth 3.5—5.5 mm *(black band partially visible, indicating pocket of 4—5 mm)*	OHI, RSD
4	Probing depth > 5.5 mm *(black band entirely within the pocket, indicating pocket of 6 mm)*	OHI, RSD. Assess the need for more complex treatment; referral to a specialist may be indicated
*	Furcation involvement	OHI, RSD. Assess the need for more complex treatment; referral to a specialist may be indicated

2.16 (a) Name four general risk factors for periodontal disease.

(b) Name two localised risk factors for periodontal disease.

(c) Give two risk factors for gingival recession.

Answer 2.16

(a) Any four of the following:
- Poor access to dental healthcare
- Smoking
- Systemic disease, eg diabetes
- Stress
- History of periodontal disease
- Genetic factors

(b) Any two of the following:
- Overhanging restorations and defective restoration margins
- Partial dentures
- Oral appliances
- Calculus

(c) Risk factors for gingival recession:
- Trauma — excessive toothbrushing, digging fingernails into gingiva, biting pencils
- Traumatic incisor relationship
- Thin tissues
- Prominent roots

2.17 (a) How does fluoride affect teeth before eruption?

(b) How does fluoride affect teeth after eruption?

(c) What are the possible consequences of fluoride overdose?

(d) What is the recommended fluoride concentration in the water supply for optimal caries prevention?

(e) What do the following terms mean and at what dose do they occur?

- Safely tolerated dose
- Potentially lethal dose
- Certainly lethal dose

Answer 2.17

(a) Effect of fluoride on teeth before eruption:
  - Teeth have more rounded cusps and shallower fissures.

  - The crystal structure of the enamel is more regular and less acid soluble.

(b) Effect of fluoride on teeth after eruption:
  - Decreases acid production by plaque bacteria

  - Prevents demineralisation and encourages remineralisation of early caries

  - Remineralised enamel is more resistant to further acid attacks

  - Thought to affect plaque and pellicle formation

(c) Possible consequences of fluoride overdose:
  - Dental effects — enamel fluorosis, mottling, pitting

  - Toxic effects — gastrointestinal

(d) 1 ppm (in UK)

(e) Terms and doses:
  - Safely tolerated dose — 1 mg/kg body weight. This is the level below which symptoms of toxicity are unlikely to occur.

  - Potentially lethal dose — 5 mg/kg body weight. This is the lowest dose that has been associated with a fatality.

  - Certainly lethal dose — 32–64 mg/kg body weight. At this dose survival of the individual is unlikely.

2.18 (a) What is pulpitis?

(b) Fill in the blanks in the following sentences using the words in the table below. You may use more than one word/phrase if you think it is appropriate.

Reversible pulpitis is a .... pain, set off by .... It is .... localised and lasts for ....

Irreversible pulpitis is a .... pain, set off by................. . It is .... localised and lasts for ....

Character	Sharp pain	Throbbing pain		
Exacerbating factors	Sweet things	Hot/cold things	Biting	Spontaneously
Localisation	Well	Poorly		
Duration	Several minutes	Several seconds	Hours	Days

(c) What types of nerve fibres are there in the pulp?

(d) What special tests could you use to help diagnose reversible/ irreversible pulpitis?

(e) What treatment is available for a tooth with irreversible pulpitis?

Answer 2.18

(a) Inflammation of the pulp

(b) Reversible pulpitis is a *sharp* pain, set off by *hot/cold things and sweet things*. It is *poorly* localised and lasts for *several seconds*. Irreversible pulpitis is a *throbbing* pain, set off by *biting or spontaneously*. It is *well* localised once the periodontal fibres are involved, and lasts for *hours*.

(c) Nerve fibre types in the pulp:
- A-β-fibres are large, fast conducting proprioceptive fibres.
- A-δ-fibres are small sensory fibres.
- C-fibres are small unmyelinated sensory fibres.

(d) Special tests:
- Percussion
- Vitality tests
- Radiographs

(e) Treatments for irreversible pulpitis:
- Root canal treatment
- Extraction

2.19 (a) Patients may have thermal sensitivity following the placement of a restoration. One theory for this is the thermal shock theory. However, another theory for the cause of thermal sensitivity is now more widely accepted — what is it called and what is it based on?

(b) How can restorative techniques limit thermal sensitivity?

(c) What are cavity sealers used for?

(d) Give the types of cavity sealer.

(e) What is meant by the term microleakage?

(f) What are the consequences of microleakage?

Answer 2.19

(a) Theory of pulpal hydrodynamics:
Fluid can move along dentinal tubules and when there is a gap between the restoration and the dentine, fluid will slowly flow outwards. A decrease in temperature leads to a sudden contraction in this fluid, and consequently increased flow, which the patient will feel as pain.

(b) When the thermal shock theory was widely accepted, insulating the cavity with a base material was used to prevent pain. Now that the hydrodynamic theory is more widely accepted the aim is to seal the dentine and increase the integrity of the interface between the dentine and the restorative material.

(c) To prevent leakage at the interface of the restorative material and the cavity walls, and to provide a protective coating to the cavity walls.

(d) Cavity sealers:
- Varnishes (eg a synthetic resin-based material or a natural resin or gum)

- Adhesive sealers which also bond at the interface between the restorative material and cavity walls (eg glass ionomer-luting cements)

(e) Microleakage is the passage of bacteria, fluids, molecules or ions along the interface of a dental restoration and the wall of the cavity preparation (Kidd, EA. *J Dent* 1976; **5**(4):199–206).

(f) Consequences of microleakage:
- Marginal discolouration of restorations

- Secondary caries

- Pulpal pathology

2.20 (a) You are cutting a cavity in a vital upper first permanent molar. You have removed all the caries but then you create a small exposure of the pulp. How would you proceed?

(b) What is this treatment called?

(c) What are you hoping will happen to the tooth by carrying out this treatment?

(d) When would this treatment not be appropriate?

(e) What are the advantages of using rubber dam for dental treatment?

Answer 2.20

(a) Management of an exposure during cavity preparation:

  1 If the tooth is not isolated already — isolate the tooth with rubber dam

  2 Dry the cavity

  3 Place calcium hydroxide over the exposure

  4 Cover with cement/liner, eg glass ionomer

  5 Restore as normal

  6 Inform the patient

  7 Arrange review

Note: there has been some work using dentine-bonding agents to cover pulpal exposures although this is not universal practice at the present time.

(b) Direct pulp capping

(c) What may happen:
  • A dentine bridge will form.

  • The pulp will remain vital.

(d) Contraindications to pulp capping:
  • Non-vital tooth

  • History of spontaneous pain — irreversible pulpitis

  • Evidence of periapical pathology

  • Large exposure

  • Contamination of the exposure with saliva, oral flora or bacteria from the caries

Also, the older the pulp the less the likelihood of success.

(e) Advantages of using rubber dam for dental treatment:
  • Isolation and moisture control — especially important for moisture sensitive techniques, eg acid etching before composite restoration

  • Prevention of inhalation of small instruments, eg during endodontic treatment

- Improved access to the tooth/teeth — no soft tissues, eg tongue in the way

- Patients do not swallow water and other irrigants

- Soft tissues protected from potentially noxious materials, eg etchant

2.21 (a) What restorative material is capable of adhesion to the tooth tissue without surface pretreatment?

(b) How may adhesion be improved?

(c) How does this material bond to tooth tissue?

(d) Besides the obvious advantage of being adherent, what other advantages are there of using this material?

(e) In what clinical situations is it used?

Answer 2.21

(a) Glass ionomer

(b) Using a polyalkenoic acid conditioner.

(c) Glass ionomer bonds by:
- Micromechanical interlocking — hybridisation of the hydroxyapatite-coated collagen fibril network

- Chemical bonding — ionic bonds form between the carboxyl groups of the polyalkenoic acid and the calcium in the hydroxyapatite

(d) Other advantages of glass ionomer:
- It releases fluoride.

- Quick to use as limited pretreatment of the tooth surface is needed.

(e) Glass ionomer is used:
- As a permanent direct restorative material, suitable for deciduous and permanent teeth

- As a temporary restoration

- As a luting cement

- As a cavity lining or base

- As a core build-up material

- As a retrograde root filling material

- As a pit and fissure sealant

2.22 (a) What do you understand by the term 'the smear layer?'

(b) Dentine can be treated with acid (or conditioned). What does this achieve?

(c) Why are primers needed during the process of creating an adhesive restoration?

(d) What do you understand by the term hybrid layer and where would you find it?

(e) What do dentine bonding agents do?

Answer 2.22

(a) When tooth tissue is cut, the debris is smeared over the tooth surface. This is called the smear layer and it contains any debris produced by reduction or instrumentation of dentine, enamel or cementum. It is calcific in nature and contaminant that precludes interaction of restorative materials with the underlying pure tooth tissue.

(b) Within dentine, acid treatment removes most of the hydroxyapatite and exposes a microporous network of collagen. The smear layer is altered or dissolved. The bonding that results is diffusion based and relies on the exposed collagen fibril scaffold being infiltrated by the resin.

(c) The dentine surface after conditioning is difficult to wet with bonding agents. The primer increases the wetability of the surface which allows the resin to spread and penetrate the tubular dentine. This improves the bonding of the subsequently applied adhesive resin.

(d) The hybrid layer is the area in which the resin of the adhesive system has interlocked with the collagen of the dentine, providing micromechanical retention.

(e) Dentine bonding agents:
   • Form resin tags in the dentinal tubules

   • Stabilise the hybrid layer

   • Form a link between the resin primer and the restorative material

2.23 (a) What are the aims of obturating a root canal?

(b) Name three causes of intra-radicular failure of a root canal treatment.

(c) Name two causes of extra-radicular failure of a root canal treatment.

(d) What are the indications for an apicectomy (surgical endodontics)?

Answer 2.23

(a) Aims of obturating a root canal:
  - To prevent reinfection of the cleaned canal
  - To prevent periradicular exudate from entering into the root canal
  - To seal any remaining bacteria in the root canal

(b) Any three of the following:
  - Necrotic material left in the canal
  - Bacteria left in the root canal system (lateral or accessory canals)
  - Contamination of the canal during treatment
  - Loss/lack of coronal seal
  - Persistent infection after treatment

(c) Two causes:
  - Root fracture
  - Radicular cysts

(d) Indications for an apicectomy:
  - Infection due to a lesion that requires a biopsy, eg radicular cyst
  - Instrument stuck in canal with residual infection
  - Impossible to fill apical third of root canal due to anatomy or pulp calcification
  - Perforation of the root
  - Post crown with excellent margins but persistent apical pathology
  - Infected, fractured apical third of root

2.24 (a) What is acid etching of enamel?

(b) What acid is commonly used and at what strength? In what form are etchants produced (eg powder, liquid) and what effect do the different forms have on working properties?

(c) How long should the acid be applied for?

(d) What do you do after applying the etchant for the above length of time?

(e) What is likely to damage the etched enamel surface and reduce the efficacy of bonding?

(f) What do you understand by the term 'total etch technique' (or etch and rinse) and which acid would you use for it?

Answer 2.24

(a) Application of a mild acid to the surface of enamel results in dissolution of about 10 μm of the surface organic component, leaving a microporous surface layer up to 50 μm deep. The surface is thus pitted, and the unfilled resin of the restorative material is able to flow into the irregularities to form resin tags that provide micromechanical retention.

(b) Phosphoric acid 30—40% is commonly used. Etchants come as gel or liquid, however, in the newer systems the etchant is combined with the dentine conditioner. The etch produced is the same with a gel or liquid but gels take twice as long to rinse away. Gels are less likely to drip onto areas where etching is not intended.

(c) Usually 15 seconds.

(d) Wash away the etchant with water for at least 15 seconds.

(e) Blood and saliva, and mechanical damage may occur by probing the area, rubbing cotton wool over it to dry it or by scraping across the surface with the suction tip or an instrument.

(f) The total etch technique involves using an acid to etch the enamel and condition the dentine at the same time. Commonly used acids include phosphoric acid (10—40%), nitric acid, maleic acid, oxalic acid and citric acid.

2.25 A 20-year-old fit and healthy woman attends your practice complaining of gaps between her upper anterior teeth. History and examination reveal that she has missing upper lateral incisors. List the treatment options in the table below. Give an advantage and disadvantage of each option. (Note: the number of rows in the table does not correspond to the exact number of treatment options, therefore all rows of the table do not have to be filled, or if you have more treatment options please write them below.)

Treatment	Advantage	Disadvantage

Answer 2.25

Treatment	Advantage	Disadvantage
Orthodontic treatment to close the spaces	No artificial teeth needed; patient does not need restorative treatment to replace the teeth	May take a long time to complete; canines may not provide a good contact against the central incisors; bleaching and restoration of the canines may be needed to make them look more like incisors and recontouring of gingival margin
Removable partial denture	Quick; cheap; does not require removal of tooth tissue (although guide planes and rests may be needed)	Not ideal for young patients; removable; in the long term will need replacing. May compromise health of gingiva/teeth if oral health /diet not ideal
Adhesive bridges	Fixed tooth in place; no or minimal preparation of abutment teeth; good aesthetics	May debond; needs favourable occlusal clearance; in the long term may need replacing
Conventional bridge	Fixed tooth in place; good aesthetics	Requires destruction of adjacent teeth; in the long term may need replacing, impairs cleansability
Implants	Permanent solution; good aesthetics; like having a 'real' tooth	Costly; may need bone grafting; requires surgery

Note: with the later four treatment options orthodontics may be required in conjunction.

2.26 (a) Name three agents that are used for chemical plaque control and state how they are thought to work.

(b) Some antimicrobials (antibiotics) have been formulated in such a way that they are suitable for use within a periodontal pocket. Give four advantages of administering a drug in this manner and name one such antimicrobial.

Answer 2.26

(a) Chemical plaque control:
- Chlorhexidine digluconate 0.12% — bacteriostatic at low doses and bacteriocidal at high concentrations. Bacterial cell walls are negatively charged due to the phosphate and carboxyl groups, but chlorhexidine is positively charged. Electrostatic charges cause the chlorhexidine to bind to the bacterial cell wall affecting the osmotic barrier and interfering with transport across the cell membrane. Unwanted effects are staining of teeth and altered taste.

- Quaternary ammonium compounds — cetylpyridinium chloride, benzalkonium chloride, benzethonium chloride. Net positive charge reacts with the negatively charged bacterial cell walls, causing disruption of the cell wall, increase in permeability and loss of the cell contents.

- Pyrimidine derivatives — hexetidine (hexahydropyridine derivative). It has antibacterial and antifungal activity, affecting the rate of ATP synthesis in bacterial mitochondria.

- Phenols — antibacterial agents that penetrate the lipid components of bacterial cell walls. These also have an anti-inflammatory action as they inhibit neutrophil chemotaxis. Examples are thymol (Listerine), bisphenol (Triclosan).

- Sanguinarine — this is a benzophenathridine alkaloid and has antibacterial properties as it causes suppression of intracellular enzymes.

- Heavy metal salts — these are thought to work by binding to the lipoteichoic acid on bacterial cell walls and altering the surface charge which in turn affects the ability of the bacteria to adhere to teeth.

- Enzymes — lactoperoxidase, hypothiocyanate. These are thought to interfere with the redox mechanism of bacterial cells.

- Surfactants — these alter the surface energy (tension) of the tooth and this interferes with plaque growth.

(b) Any four of the following:
- Drug is actually delivered to where it is needed, not throughout the whole body.

- High local drug concentrations can be achieved.

- There are fewer systemic side effects.

- Overall lower doses of the drug need to be administered.

- Drug delivery is not dependent on patient compliance.

- There is prolonged drug release.

    Example — any one of the following:

- Antimicrobials

- Tetracycline

- Metronidazole

2.27 (a) What is a composite restorative material?

(b) List the types of composite restorative material you know in the table below. Give an advantage/disadvantage of each type.

Material	Advantage	Disadvantage

(c) After placing a composite restoration how do you finish and polish it?

Answer 2.27

(a) It is a type of restorative material made of a mixture of materials (hence the name): organic resin matrix, an inorganic filler and a coupling agent

(b)

Material	Advantage	Disadvantage
Traditional composites	Good mechanical properties	Surface roughness; difficult to polish
Microfilled resins	Very good surface polish	Poor wear resistance; unsuitable for load-bearing areas; high contraction shrinkage
Hybrid (blended) composites	Good mechanical properties; good surface polish	
Small particle hybrid composites	Good mechanical properties; very good surface polish	

(c) Finishing involves shaping and smoothing the restoration to the anatomical form and polishing imparts a shine to the surface. The smoothest surface is achieved when composite is polymerised against an acetate strip with no polishing. This however, leaves a surface with a very high resin content that is not resistant to wear. For polishing:

- Diamond and carbide burs are used for gross finishing.

- Rubber cups with abrasive materials of differing coarseness. The coarsest ones are used for gross finishing and the finer ones for polishing. They are good in areas with irregularities and the lingual surface of anterior teeth.

- Flexible abrasive discs.

- Finishing strips for interproximal areas

2.28 (a) What are the risk factors for developing root caries?

(b) How would you manage a patient with multiple root caries?

(c) What restorative materials are commonly used for class V lesions?

Answer 2.28

(a) Risk factors of root caries:
- Exposure of the root surface (pocketing, gingival recession or attachment loss)
- Cariogenic diet
- Decreased salivary flow (medications, previous radiotherapy, drugs, diabetes, ageing)
- Poor oral hygiene — inaccessible areas (eg periodontal pockets); decreased manual dexterity; lack of access to dental healthcare or dental health is a low priority; removable prosthesis; restorations

(b) Elimination of active infection (remove caries and place restorations), and preventive measures:

1 Identify any risk factors that can be corrected

2 Oral hygiene advice

3 Dietary analysis and advice

4 Periodontal treatment as necessary

5 Fluoride treatment in the surgery (eg Duraphat application) or home application (eg rinses)

6 Recall

(c) Glass ionomer, resin-modified glass ionomer, composite and amalgam.

2.29 (a) It is possible to bond amalgam to tooth structure. Give four potential advantages of this over non-bonded restorations of amalgam.

(b) What other restorative materials can be bonded to tooth tissue?

(c) If you wanted to bond materials that are commonly used for anterior crowns how would they be pre-treated?

Answer 2.29

(a) Any four of the following:
- Decrease in microleakage — less destructive of tooth tissue as traditional methods of creating retention for restorations involve removing tooth tissue to create dovetails, undercuts and grooves, etc
- May limit the need for dentine pins
- May increase fracture resistance of restored teeth
- Transmits and distributes force better
- There may be less postoperative sensitivity due to better sealing of the margins.

(b) Materials that can be bonded to tooth tissue:
- Glass ionomers
- Composites
- Hybrid restorative materials, eg resin-modified glass ionomers, compomers
- Ceramics — using special cements

(c) Pre-treatment of anterior crowns:
- Conventional ceramics that are silica based are treated with hydrofluoric acid and ammonium bifluoride. They may also be sandblasted or air abraded. They are often treated with silane coupling agents.
- Alumina and zirconium oxide ceramics are surface roughened with air abrasion and then the surface is coated with a silicate.

2.30 (a) What materials are commonly used for primary impressions for complete dentures?

(b) What broad groups can hydrocolloid impression materials and synthetic elastomeric impression materials be divided into?

(c) What do you understand by the following terms. Give one disadvantage of each.

- Mucostatic impression

- Mucocompressive impression

(d) What do you understand by the term selective mucocompressive impression?

Answer 2.30

(a) Materials for primary impressions:
  - Alginate

  - Compound — thermoplastic

  - Impression putty

(b) Hydrocolloids can be divided into: reversible (agar) and irreversible (alginate). Synthetic elastomeric impression materials can be divided into:
  - Elastomers

  - Polysulphides

  - Polyethers

  - Silicones (addition cured/condensation cured)

(c) A mucostatic impression is an impression taken with the mucosa in its resting state. It provides a good fit at rest and therefore good retention, ie most of the time but when the patient chews the denture will tend to rock around the most incompressible areas, eg a palatine torus. A mucocompressive impression is an impression taken when the denture-bearing area is subjected to compressive force. This results in a denture that is maximally stable during function but not at rest.

(d) This is an impression taken with only certain areas of the denture-bearing area being subjected to the compressive force.

2.31 (a) What is meant by the terms RVD and OVD and what is their significance?

(b) Name one way of measuring the RVD or the OVD.

(c) In which patients is it important to measure the OVD?

(d) What factors may affect the jaw position at rest?

Answer 2.31

(a) RVD is resting vertical dimension. It is a measure of the vertical height of the patient's lower face and is measured as the distance between two arbitrary points — one related to the maxilla and the other to the mandible with the patient at rest. OVD is the occlusal vertical dimension. It is a similar measure to that mentioned above, but is taken with the patient's teeth in occlusion. The difference between the two measurements gives the freeway space, which is the vertical gap between the patient's teeth at rest.

(b) Any one of the following:
- Willis gauge to measure between two points on the face (eg nose and chin)

- Willis gauge to measure between the pupil of the eye and the mouth and then compare this with the distance between the base of the nose and the inferior border of the chin

- Using two dots on two points on the face (eg nose and chin)

- Swallowing, which is thought to show the rest vertical dimension

- Phonetic methods

- Appearance

(c) Those patients with partial dentures and no natural teeth occluding, and patients with complete dentures or when changing the OVD of a worn dentition.

(d) What factors may affect the rest jaw position?
- Stress

- Head posture

- Pain

- Age

- Neuromuscular disorders

- Bruxism

2.32 (a) What do you understand by the following terms:

- Group function

- Canine guidance

- Balanced occlusion

(b) Which would you try to create in a complete denture case?

(c) What is the difference between balanced occlusion and balanced articulation?

(d) When trying to achieve the correct occlusion in a complete denture case what factors will affect the occlusion in protrusive movements?

(e) What do you understand by the term lateral compensating curve and how does it affect the set up of complete denture teeth?

Answer 2.32

(a) Group function means that during lateral excursions there is contact between several upper and lower teeth on the working side and no contacts on the non-working side. Canine guidance means that during lateral excursions there is contact between upper and lower canine teeth on the working side only and no contact on the non-working side. Balanced occlusion means simultaneous contacts between opposing artificial teeth on both sides of the dental arch.

(b) Balanced occlusion

(c) Balanced articulation is simultaneous contact of opposing teeth in central and eccentric positions as the mandible moves, ie it is a dynamic relationship whereas balanced occlusion is a static situation.

(d) Factors affecting the occlusion in protrusive movements:
- Incisor guidance angle
- Cusp angles of the posterior teeth
- Condylar guidance angles
- Orientation of the occlusal plane
- Prominence of the compensating curve

(e) During lateral excursions the mandible does not move in a horizontal plane only. There are vertical components to the movement due to the condylar guidance angle and the incisor guidance angle. To achieve occlusion in lateral excursions when the mandible and lower denture carry out these tipping movements the upper teeth need to be inclined buccally so that the occlusal planes of the teeth lie on a curve (viewed in the coronal plane). This is analogous to the Monson curve in the natural dentition.

2.33 (a) Give three advantages and three disadvantages of an immediate denture.

(b) What do the terms flanged and open face mean with respect to an immediate upper complete denture? Give an advantage and disadvantage of each.

(c) If you wanted to adjust the fit of an immediate denture in the future what methods can you use?

Answer 2.33

(a) Advantages — any three of the following:
- Patient is never without teeth and so there are psychological advantages.
- Aesthetics — patient is never without teeth.
- Artificial teeth can be set in the same position as the natural ones.
- Soft tissue support
- Easier to register jaw relations as they are taken when the patient had teeth.
- Bleeding easier to control after extractions

Disadvantages — any three of the following:
- Denture may not fit after extraction.
- Will need relining/copying or remaking.
- Will not fit when the alveolus remodels
- Unable to try-in.
- May need many visits for adjustment.

(b) Flanged means that the denture has a flanged periphery, like a normal complete denture. The advantage is that retention is good and will make future adjustments easier. The disadvantage is that the lip may be over supported/appear too bulbous. Open faced means that there is no buccal flange and the denture teeth sit at the edge of the extraction sockets of the natural teeth. The advantage is that it can be used when there are large undercuts, it often has good aesthetics initially, but the retention is poor and when resorption occurs a gap appears between the gingival margin of the denture teeth and the mucosa.

(c) Methods to adjust the fit of an immediate denture:
- Relining
- Rebasing
- Copy dentures
- Total remake

2.34   What is meant by the term altered cast technique? Explain the theory behind it. What stages are involved in carrying it out and in what situation could you use it?

Answer 2.34

When a patient wears a denture with a free end saddle(s) (FES) supported by both tooth and soft tissue there is a risk that when a load is applied to the saddle (eg during function) the underlying mucosa will compress and the saddle will move. The part of the denture supported by the teeth will only move as much as the periodontal ligament of the teeth moves and so this differential movement will cause the denture to rotate. To overcome this an impression of the FES area is taken with the mucosa compressed so that minimal displacement will occur with loading and this reduces the rotation effect. However, overcompression of the soft tissues must be avoided as this can lead to either displacement of the denture when the tissues try to recover or to pressure necrosis of the mucosa.

This technique of taking a special mucocompressive impression of just the FES area(s) is known as the altered cast technique (of Applegate). The idea is to compensate for the difference in degree of support offered by the mucosa and the teeth.

Method:

1 The denture framework has base plates attached to the FES area. These are relieved to allow about 2 mm of space between them and the mucosa.

2 An impression is taken of the FES area with pressure applied only to the tooth supported part of the denture and no pressure applied over the FES.

3 The original working master cast is sectioned to remove the FES area.

4 The denture framework is reseated on to the cast and the FES impression area cast up.

2.35 (a) What is a dental surveyor and what is the objective of surveying the diagnostic cast?

(b) What is a dental articulator?

(c) How would you classify articulators?

(d) What is a facebow and what is it used for?

Answer 2.35

(a) A dental surveyor is an instrument that is used to determine the relative parallelism of two or more surfaces of the teeth or other parts of the cast of a dental arch. The objectives of surveying the diagnostic cast are to identify:

- The most desirable path of insertion that will eliminate or minimise interference to placement and removal

- Tooth and tissue undercuts

- Tooth surfaces that are, or need to be, parallel so that they act as guide planes during insertion and removal

- And measure areas of teeth that may be used for retention

- Whether tooth and bony areas of interference need to be eliminated surgically by selecting different paths of insertion

- Undesirable tooth undercut that needs to be avoided, blocked out or eliminated

- Potential sites for occlusal rests and where they need to be prepared

(b) It is an instrument that is used to reproduce jaw relationships and movements of the lower jaw relative to the upper. Casts of both upper and lower jaws are mounted on the articulator.

(c) Classification of articulators:
- Hinge articulator

- Average value articulator

- Adjustable articulator — simple adjustable; fully adjustable

(d) A facebow is an instrument that measures the relationship of either the maxillary or mandibular arch to the intercondylar axis and is used to transfer these measurements to an articulator. This means that the articulated casts will have the same relationship to the hinge axis of the articulator as the teeth with the intercondylar axis.

2.36 (a) Name five muscles, the movements of which may affect the peripheral flanges of a complete denture.

(b) Where is the posterior margin of an upper complete denture usually situated?

- Anterior to the fovea palatinae

- Posterior to the fovea palatinae

(c) What is a post-dam and what function does it perform?

(d) Where is it usually positioned?

(e) What do you understand by the term 'neutral zone?'

Answer 2.36

(a) Any five of the following:
 - Geniohyoid

 - Orbicularis oris

 - Mentalis

 - Mylohyoid

 - Buccinator

 - Palatopharyngeus

 - Palatoglossus

(b) Location of the posterior margin of the upper complete denture:
 - Anterior to the fovea palatinae

(c) A post-dam is a raised lip on the posterior border of the fit surface of an upper complete denture. It compresses the palatal soft tissue to form a border seal.

(d) It usually lies at the junction of the non-moveable hard palate (anteriorly) and the moveable soft palate (posteriorly).

(e) The area between the tongue, lips and cheeks where the displacing forces of the muscles is minimal. It is the ideal area into which a prosthesis should be placed to minimise displacing forces.

2.37 (a) What is the Kennedy classification for partially edentulous arches?

(b) What Kennedy classification does this charting fit into?

4321	123
54321	12347

(c) What are the stages in designing a partial denture?

(d) What is meant by the term direct retainer in a partial denture?

(e) Name the two broad classes of clasps.

(f) Clasps do not work in isolation, but are often termed as being part of a clasp unit. What else is incorporated into a clasp unit?

(g) Why are these other features needed?

Answer 2.37

(a) Kennedy classification:
- Class I — bilateral edentulous areas located posterior to the natural teeth
- Class II — unilateral edentulous areas located posterior to the remaining natural teeth
- Class III — a unilateral edentulous area with natural teeth remaining both anterior and posterior (bounded saddle)
- Class IV — a single, but bilateral (crossing the midline) edentulous area located anterior to the remaining natural teeth

Once the classification has been decided each additional edentulous gap is indicated by a modification number. Class IV does not have modifications.

(b) Example classification:
- Upper — Kennedy class I
- Lower — Kennedy class II modification 1

(c) Stages in designing a partial denture:
1 Outline the saddle areas

2 Place occlusal rests seats

3 Place clasps for direct retention

4 Place the indirect retainers

5 Connect the denture

(d) Any element of a partial denture that provides resistance to movement of the denture away from the supporting tissues is a direct retainer.

(e) Clasps may be:
- Gingivally approaching
- Occlusally approaching

(f) A clasp unit also has:
- Some form of support, usually an occlusal rest.
- Some form of reciprocation.

(g) Support will allow loads to be transferred along the long axis of teeth. It will also enable the clasp arm to be accurately located in the undercut on the tooth. Reciprocation is needed as all clasps on teeth must be balanced by something on the opposite surface to act as a balance. This will prevent inadvertent force being applied to a tooth in one direction only and acting like an orthodontic appliance.

2.38 (a) Copy dentures are sometimes indicated for patients. In what situations would these be made?

(b) What are the advantages of making a set of copy dentures?

(c) Briefly describe the stages in making a set of copy dentures.

Answer 2.38

(a) Indications for copy dentures:
- Occlusal wear on a set of previously successful complete dentures.
- Need for replacement of the denture base material.
- Patient was initially given immediate dentures and they need to be replaced.
- Patient has a set of complete dentures that they have been happy with but are now unretentive/worn, especially elderly patients who may find it hard to adapt to a completely new set of dentures.
- To make a spare set of dentures.
- If a patient has had problems with previous dentures it is advisable to copy the set that they like the most.

(b) Advantages:
- Simple clinical steps, quicker than starting from scratch.
- Reduced number of laboratory steps: no special trays needed; no record blocks needed.
- Patient is never without their denture.
- Original dentures are not altered in any way.
- More predictable patient acceptance.

(c) Steps for making copy dentures (one method — others are available):
1 Alginate impressions are taken of the dentures in boxes.

2 The dentures are given back to the patient.

3 In the lab the alginate moulds are poured up in self-curing acrylic bases.

4 The copy dentures are now assessed and adjusted as necessary by the clinician and tried in the patient's mouth and used to take an occlusal record.

5 These are sent to the laboratory and articulated, and then denture teeth are set up.

6 The copy dentures are used as special trays and impressions are taken of the fit surface.

7 In the laboratory the copy dentures are converted into heat-cured acrylic dentures.

2.39 (a)   Fill in the blanks from the following list of words:

.... is tooth surface loss from non-bacterial .... attack. Smooth
.... surfaces are seen with restorations standing .... Tooth surface
loss of the .... surfaces of the .... incisors is seen in cases of gastric
reflux and vomiting. .... is physical wear of a tooth by an external agent
and may result in .... cavities at the .... is physical wear
of a tooth by another tooth, and it commonly affects .... and ....
surfaces. Abfraction lesions are thought to be due to a combination of
.... and occlusally-induced tooth ....

1   erosion/attrition/abrasion

2   mechanical/chemical/thermal

3   plaque free/plaque covered

4   low/proud/level

5   buccal/palatal/interproximal

6   lower/upper

7   class III/class IV/class V

8   gingival margins/occlusal edges/palatal surfaces

9   flexure/wear/caries

(b)   What could be the cause of severe erosion in a 16-year-old girl?

(c)   What specialist treatment should she receive?

Answer 2.39

(a) *Erosion* is tooth surface loss from non-bacterial *chemical* attack. Smooth *plaque-free* surfaces are seen with restorations standing *proud*. Tooth surface loss of the *palatal* surfaces of the upper incisors is seen in cases of gastric reflux and vomiting. *Abrasion* is physical wear of a tooth by an external agent and may result in *class V* cavities at the *gingival margins*. *Attrition* is physical wear of a tooth by another tooth, and it commonly affects *occlusal* and *interproximal* surfaces. Abfraction lesions are thought to be due to a combination of *abrasion* and occlusally-induced tooth *flexure*.

(b) Vomiting — bulimia nervosa; less likely — gastric reflux or pregnancy. Most likely excessive fizzy drinks/cola consumption.

(c) If you suspect that she has bulimia nervosa then that is outside the scope of management for a dental practitioner. She needs to be referred to her general/medical practitioner for further assessment and possible referral on to a psychiatrist.

2.40 (a) You need to carry out root canal treatment on a mandibular first permanent molar and a maxillary first permanent molar.

On the given diagrams of the occlusal surfaces of these teeth, mark where you will expect to find the root canals.

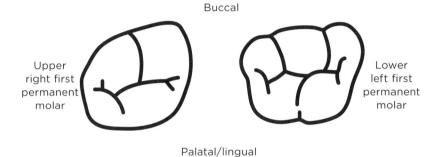

Buccal

Upper right first permanent molar

Lower left first permanent molar

Palatal/lingual

(b) How can you determine the working length of a root canal?

(c) What do you understand by the terms zip, elbow and transportation with respect to preparation of root canals?

Answer 2.40

(a)

Black dots represent root canals — four in the
upper molar and three in the lower molar

(b) With the use of:
   - An apex locator

   - Working length radiograph with an instrument in the canal

(c) Zip and elbow are phenomena that occur due to instruments trying to straighten out within a root canal. An hourglass shape is created with the narrowest part being called the elbow and the zip being the flared apical part. The problem with this type of canal shape is that it is difficult to fill the apical portion well. Transportation is the selective removal of dentine from one area of the root canal. This is done electively, for example when widening the coronal part of a root canal, or it can be an iatrogenic error.

2.41 (a) What are the advantages of using a crown down method for preparation of a root canal?

(b) Why are root canals irrigated during preparation for root canal filling?

(c) Name two commonly used irrigants.

(d) Give five properties of an ideal root canal-filling material.

Answer 2.41

(a) Preparing the canal from the crown down gives better access. Flaring of the coronal part first removes restrictions and helps prevent instruments binding short of the working length. The coronal part is usually where most of the infected material is present. If this is removed and cleaned first it limits the possibility of spreading the infected material to the apical and periapical tissues. If you estimate the working length and then change the coronal part of the preparation it may inadvertently alter the length. Coronal preparation first allows irrigants to gain access to more of the root canal system.

(b) Physical removal of dentine by instruments does not get rid of all the bacteria in the root canal system. Irrigants reach the areas instruments cannot, and remove bacteria that would otherwise be inaccessible.

(c) Any two of the following:
- Sodium hypochlorite
- EDTA (ethylenediaminetetraacetic acid)
- Local anaesthetic solution
- Chlorhexidine
- Iodine-based irrigant
- Citric acid

(d) Any five of the following:
- It must be capable of sealing the canal apically, laterally and coronally.
- It should be radiopaque.
- It should be bacteriostatic.
- It should not irritate the periradicular tissues.
- It should be easy to handle, insert and if necessary remove.
- It should be impervious to moisture.
- It should be dimensionally stable.

2.42 (a) What is an overdenture and how does it differ from an onlay denture?

(b) Give four advantages of an overdenture.

(c) In what groups of patients would overdentures be useful?

(d) What factors need to be considered in choosing and preparing the abutment teeth?

Answer 2.42

(a) An overdenture is a denture which derives its support from one or more abutment teeth by completely covering them beneath its fitting surface. An onlay denture is a partial denture that overlays the occlusal surface of all or some of the teeth. It is often used to increase the occlusal vertical dimension.

(b) Any four of the following:
- Preservation of the alveolar bone around the retained roots
- Improved stability, retention and support
- Preserved proprioception
- Decreased crown:root ratio which reduces damaging lateral forces and reduces mobility in teeth with reduced periodontal support
- Increased masticatory force
- Psychological benefit of not losing all teeth

(c) Overdentures are useful in:
- Severe tooth wear
- Patients with hypodontia
- Cleft lip and palate patients
- Motivated patients with good oral hygiene

(d) Factors to consider:
- The abutment should ideally be bilateral and symmetrical with a minimum of one tooth space between them.
- Order of preference: canine, molars, premolars, incisors
- Healthy attached gingivae and periodontal support, minimal mobility
- Dome root surface 2–4 mm above gingival margin
- Root canal treatment may be required.

2.43 (a) What is the definition of osseointegration?

(b) Give three situations when implants may be used in the head and neck.

(c) Give three patient-related factors that may affect the success of implant placement.

(d) What anatomical factors need to be considered with regard to implant placement?

(e) What would you see clinically if an implant failed?

(f) Success rate for single tooth implants are .... than in edentulous patients. Success rate for implants in partially dentate patients are .... than in edentulous patients. Choose the correct answer from the following: better, comparable, worse.

Answer 2.43

(a) A direct structural and functional union between ordered living bone and the surface of a load-carrying implant (Albrektsson T, Brånemark PI, Hansson HA, Lindström J. Osteointegrated titanium implants. Requirements for ensuring a long-lasting, direct bone anchorage in man. *Acra Orthop Scand* 1981; **52**:155–170).

(b) Any three of the following:
- Single tooth replacement
- Bridge abutment
- Support for overdentures
- To support facial prosthesis and hearing aids
- Orthodontic anchorage

(c) Any three of the following:
- Oral hygiene
- Periodontal disease
- Previous radiotherapy
- Smoking
- Bisphosphonate medication and anti-resorptive/anti-angiogenesis drug usage

(d) Anatomical factors:
- Bone height
- Bone width
- Bone density or quality
- Proximity of inferior dental nerve
- Proximity of maxillary sinus
- Tooth position

(e) Clinical features of a failed implant:
- Mobility

- Pain

- Ongoing marginal bone loss

- Soft tissue infection

- Peri-implantitis

(f) Success rate for single tooth implants are *better* than in edentulous patients. Success rate for implants in partially dentate patients are *better* than in edentulous patients (Esposito M, Hirsch J-M, Lekholm U, Thomsen P. Biological factors contributing to failures of osseointergrated oral implants. *Eur J Oral Sci* 1998; **106**:527–551).

2.44 (a) What are the constituents of dental amalgam?

(b) What are the γ, γ^1 and γ^2 phases, and what is the importance of these different phases?

(c) What is the setting reaction of dental amalgam?

(d) What do you understand by the terms lathe cut particles and spherical particles? What is the significance of the different types?

(e) Why is it common practice to overfill a cavity and then carve it down?

(f) How should do you store waste amalgam?

Answer 2.44

(a) Constituents of dental amalgam:
- Silver
- Tin
- Copper
- Zinc
- Mercury

(b) Gamma (γ) phase is Ag_3Sn; γ^1 phase is Ag_2Hg_3; and γ^2 phase is Sn_7Hg. The γ^2 phase is the weakest part of the amalgam — it has the lowest tensile strength and is the softest of the phases. If the amount of γ^2 phase can be limited in the final dental amalgam the resulting amalgam will be stronger.

(c) $Ag_3Sn + Hg = Ag_3Sn + Ag_2Hg_3 + Sn_7Hg$
$(\gamma + \text{mercury} = \gamma + \gamma_1 + \gamma_2)$

This is followed by $\gamma_2 + AgCu \rightarrow Cu_6Sn_5 + \gamma_1$: leaving little or no γ_2.

(d) Lathe cut alloy is made by chipping off pieces from a solid ingot of the alloy. This results in particles of different shapes and sizes. Spherical particles are made by melting the ingredients of the alloy together and spraying them into an inert atmosphere. The droplets then solidify into spherical pellets that are regular in shape and can be more closely packed together. This results in amalgam that requires less condensation force and results in increased strength of the amalgam.

(e) When amalgam is condensed the mercury rises to the surface of the restoration. To try to minimise the residual mercury left in the restoration it is usual to overfill the preparation and the excess mercury-rich amalgam can be carved away leaving the lower mercury containing amalgam which has a greater strength and better longevity.

(f) In a sealed container under liquid, usually X-ray fixative, solution.

2.45 (a) What are dental ceramics made out of?

(b) What are the three technical stages in producing a porcelain jacket crown?

(c) Give one advantage and disadvantage of porcelain jacket crowns.

(d) How has the main disadvantage of porcelain jacket crowns been overcome?

(e) What does CAD-CAM mean in connection with ceramic restorations?

(f) Give three requirements of a metal-ceramic alloy.

Answer 2.45

(a) Ceramics are made of feldspar, silica (quartz) and kaolin.

(b) The first stage is compaction. The powder is mixed with water and applied to the die so as to remove as much water as possible and compact the material such that there is a high density of particles, which minimises firing shrinkage. The next stage is firing. The crown is heated in a furnace to allow the molten glass to flow between the powder particles and fill the voids. The last stage is glazing, which is done to produce a smooth and impervious outer layer.

(c) Advantages — any one of the following:
  • Excellent aesthetics

  • Low thermal conductivity

  • High resistance to wear

  • Glazed surface resists plaque accumulation

  Disadvantages — any one of the following:
  • Poor strength and very brittle, so often fracture

  • Firing shrinkage so must be overbuilt

(d) By fusing the porcelain to metal to produce metal ceramic restorations, by making reinforced ceramic core systems and by creating resin-bonded ceramics.

(e) Computer-assisted/aided design, computer-assisted/aided manufacture.

(f) Any three of the following:
  • High bond strength to the ceramic

  • No adverse reaction with the ceramic

  • Melting temperature must be greater than the firing temperature of the ceramic

  • Accurate fit

  • Biocompatible

  • No corrosion

  • Easy to use and cast

  • High elastic modulus

  • Low cost

2.46 (a) What are the uses of dental cements?

(b) Give two examples of the types of material used for each purpose.

(c) Which zinc-based cement bonds to tooth substance?

(d) How should this material be mixed and why?

(e) Which cement should not be used under composite restorations and why?

(f) Which material is used for pulp capping and why?

(g) Which cement is thought to reduce sensitivity of a deep restoration?

Answer 2.46

(a) Uses of dental cements:
- Luting agents
- Cavity linings and bases
- Temporary restorations

(b) Examples:
- Luting agents — modified zinc phosphate, zinc oxide and eugenol, zinc polycarboxylate, glass ionomer, resin modified glass ionomer, compomers, resin cements
- Cavity linings and bases — calcium hydroxide, zinc oxide and eugenol
- Temporary restorations — zinc oxide and eugenol, glass ionomer

(c) Zinc polycarboxylate.

(d) On a glass slab as it must not be mixed on anything that absorbs water, also a glass slab can be cooled and this will increase the working time.

(e) Zinc oxide and eugenol as the eugenol is thought to interfere with the proper setting of the composite material.

(f) Calcium hydroxide as it is extremely alkaline (pH 11), which helps with formation of reparative dentine. It is also antibacterial and has a long duration of action.

(g) Zinc oxide and eugenol is thought to reduce sensitivity due to the obtundent and analgesic properties of the eugenol.

2.47 (a) What are the indications for anterior veneers?

(b) What materials are used for veneers?

(c) What would you need to check prior to advising placement of veneers?

(d) What is the long term prognosis of veneers and what would you warn the patient about?

(e) What is the thickness of the veneers?

(f) What are the key points during tooth preparation?

Answer 2.47

(a) Indications for anterior veneers:
  - Discolouration of teeth
  - For closure of spaces/midline diastema
  - Hypoplastic teeth
  - Fracture of teeth
  - Modifying the shape of a tooth

(b) Materials used:
  - Porcelain
  - Composite (direct/indirect)

(c) Check the following:
  - Is the discolouration enough to warrant treatment or is it so severe that it will not be masked?
  - The patient's smile line — this helps to determine which teeth need treatment for aesthetic reasons only and also the position of the cervical margin
  - Is there enough crown present to support a veneer?
  - Any occlusal restrictions, eg edge to edge occlusion, imbrication?
  - Any parafunctional activities?
  - Is there an alternative option, eg bleaching?

(d) May require replacement in the long term (eg approximately 4 years for composite veneers) as a result of:
  - Risk of chipping of incisal edge
  - Debonding
  - Need to keep good gingival health

(e) Usually 0.5–0.7 mm

(f) Key points during tooth preparation:
  - Tooth reduction labially — depth cuts are helpful.

  - Chamfer finish line is helpful for the technician.

  - Margin — slightly supragingival unless discolouration, then margin can be subgingival.

  - Extend into embrasure but short of contact point.

  - Incisally either chamfer or wrap over onto palatal surface.

2.48 (a) What is the function of a post and core?

(b) What is important to check prior to placement of a post and why?

(c) What is the ideal length of the post?

(d) Give a classification of a post and core system.

(e) What are the ideal characteristics of a post?

(f) What measures can be taken to avoid post perforation?

(g) How would you manage a post perforation?

Answer 2.48

(a) Provides support and retention for the restoration and distributes stresses along the root.

(b) The condition of the orthograde root filling and the apical condition as placement of the post will make it difficult to redo the root canal filling so if necessary repeat orthograde root canal treatment.

(c) Ideal length is at least the length of the crown; approximately two-thirds of the canal length; and the apical seal must not be disturbed so at least 4 mm of well-condensed gutta percha should be left.

(d) Classification of post and core system:
   • Prefabricated or custom made
   • Parallel sided or tapered
   • Threaded, smooth or serrated

(e) A post should:
   • Have adequate length
   • Be as parallel as possible
   • Have a roughened or serrated surface
   • Not rotate in the root canal

(f) Careful choice of post:
   • Avoid large diameter post in small tapered roots, instead used tapered post and cement passively
   • Avoid long post in curved roots
   • Avoid threaded post which will increase internal stress within root canal

(g) Depends on the location of the perforation. If it is in the coronal third try to incorporate into the design of the post crown, eg diaphragm post and core preparation. For a minimal perforation in the middle third, seal the perforation (eg lateral condensation) and reposition the post. For a perforation in the apical two-thirds, use a surgical approach to try to reduce the exposed post and seal the perforation. If attempting repair of perforations, the use of MTA — mineral trioxide aggregate — would be preferable. Due to the poor long-term prognosis, extraction and implant placement may be favoured.

2.49 (a) When are posterior crowns used?

(b) What are the principles of tooth preparation for a posterior crown?

(c) How much tooth reduction is required for different materials used for posterior crowns?

(d) What features affect the retention and resistance form of the crown preparation? Give three for each form.

(e) What are the advantages of partial coverage crown over full coverage crown?

Answer 2.49

(a) Post crowns are used for:
- Bridge abutments.
- Restoring endodontically treated teeth.
- Repairing tooth substance lost due to extensive caries/remaining tooth substance requires protection.
- Fractured teeth.
- Situations in which it is difficult to produce a reasonable occlusal form in a plastic material.

(b) Principles of tooth preparation:
- Remove enough tooth substance to allow adequate thickness of material (see below).
- Develop adequate retention and resistance form.
- Marginal integrity, supragingival and onto sound tooth where possible.

(c) Tooth reduction required:
- Full veneer gold crown — 1.5 mm on functional cusp, 1 mm elsewhere.
- Porcelain fused to metal crown — same tooth reduction as for gold crown except where porcelain coverage is required where more tooth substance must be removed.
- Occlusal reduction — metal occlusal surface requires same tooth reduction as for gold crown.
- All porcelain — occlusal surface 2 mm supporting cusps and 1.5 mm non-supporting cusps; buccal reduction 1.2–1.5 mm; margins 1.2–1.5 mm; shoulder: if porcelain to tooth margin otherwise chamfer finish as for gold crown.

(d) Retention relies on the height, diameter and taper of the preparation. It will also be increased by the placement of boxes, groves, pins and surface texture. Resistance relies on taper of preparation, height to diameter ratio, correctly aligned and positioned grooves and boxes.

(e) Advantages of partial coverage crown:
  - Preservation of tooth structure
  - Less pulpal damage
  - Margins more likely to be supragingival
  - Remaining tooth substance can act as a guide for the technician

2.50 (a) A 21-year-old woman presents with gingival recession affecting the lower incisors. How will you manage this?

(b) If the recession is mild on all except the lower left lateral incisor how would you proceed?

(c) What are the possible causes of gingival recession?

(d) If the gingival recession continues on the lower left lateral incisor what other options may you consider?

(e) If a graft is considered to treat a defect such as that mentioned in (d), where would it be taken from?

Answer 2.50

(a) Take a thorough history:
- Present concerns, sensitivity
- History of presenting complaint
- Dental history
- Toothbrushing history, frequency and duration
- Any previous orthodontic treatment

Then examination should include assessment of presence of plaque, recession, probing depth, bleeding, amount of attached gingivae, presence of functional gingivae, tooth mobility, vitality testing, occlusion, oral hygiene technique and instructions.

(b) Target traumatic tooth brushing and improve plaque control; monitor the progression with clinical measurements, photographs; and treat sensitivity. Take impression for study models.

(c) Causes of gingival recession:
- Traumatic toothbrushing
- Incorrect toothbrushing technique
- Abrasive toothpaste
- Traumatic occlusion/incisor relationship
- Tooth out of line of arch
- Orthodontic movement of tooth labially
- Habits such as rubbing of gingivae with fingernail, pen, etc.

(d) Mucogingival surgery to correct recession by a:
- Lateral pedicle graft
- Double papilla flap
- Coronally repositioned flap (these can be sewn with a interpositional graft)
- Free gingival graft to provide a wider and functional zone of attached gingivae
- Thin acrylic gingival veneer/stent (rarely used)

(e) Palate

2.51 (a) Give six clinical features of necrotising ulcerative gingivitis.

(b) What organisms are implicated?

(c) What are the risk factors for necrotising ulcerative gingivitis?

(d) How would you treat it?

Answer 2.51

(a) Any six of the following:
- Painful yellowish white ulcer
- Initially involve the interdental papillae
- Spread to involve the labial and lingual marginal gingivae
- Metallic taste
- Regional lymphadenopathy
- Fever
- Malaise
- Poor oral hygiene
- Sensation of teeth being wedged apart
- Fetor oris

(b) Mixed picture: fuso-spirochaetal organisms (*Borrelia vincentii*, *Fusobacterium fusiformis*) and Gram-negative anaerobes including *Porphyromonas*, *Treponema* species, *Selenomonas* species and *Prevotella* species.

(c) Risk factors are:
- Poor oral hygiene
- Pre-existing gingivitis
- Smoking
- Stress
- Malnourishment and debilitation
- Human immunodeficiency virus (HIV) infection

(d) Treatment of necrotising ulcerative gingivitis:
- Local measures
- Oral hygiene instruction
- Debridement
- Chemical plaque control, eg chlorhexidine

- Metronidazole 200–400 mg three times daily for 3 days if systemically unwell

- Advice on management of risk factors, oral hygiene instruction, nutritional advice

2.52 (a) How can you classify periodontal disease?

(b) Define localised aggressive periodontitis.

(c) How do you manage it?

(d) Give four indications for periodontal surgery.

Answer 2.52

(a) Gingival disease:
   - Gingivitis

   - Necrotising ulcerative gingivitis (NUG)

   Periodontal disease:
   - (Aggressive periodontitis) Early onset periodontitis (prepubertal, juvenile periodontitis)

   - (Aggressive periodontitis) Rapidly progressive periodontitis

   - Adult periodontitis

   - Necrotising ulcerative periodontitis

   - HIV periodontitis

   Alternative classification of periodontal disease (Armitage GC, 1999, British Society Periodontology, Young Practitioners Guide to Periodontology 2012, www.bsperio.org.uk)
   - I — Chronic periodontitis

   - II — Aggressive periodontitis

   - III — Periodontitis as a manifestation of systemic disease

   - IV — Necrotising periodontal disease

   - V — Abscesses of the periodontium

   - VI — Periodontitis associated with endodontic lesions

   - VII — Development of acquired deformities and conditions

(b) An aggressive periodontitis occurring in an otherwise healthy adolescence, characterised by rapid loss of connective tissue attachment and alveolar bone loss. Usually localised to the incisors and first molars although it can be generalised.

(c) Management of localised aggressive periodontitis:

   1 Oral hygiene instruction

   2 MCS (microbiology culture and sensitivity) of subgingival flora

   3 Scale and root surface debridement and/or access flap surgery

   4 Antibiotics (usually responds to tetracycline)

   5 Consider surgical excision of pocket lining

(d) There are no strict indications of periodontal surgery but in certain clinical situations it is more likely to be indicated:

   - Pockets greater than 6 mm

   - Pockets associated with thick fibrous gingivae

   - Furcation involvement

   - Mucogingival deformities or extensive periodontitis lesion requiring reconstruction or regenerative treatment

   - Short clinical crown requiring increase in clinical crown height

   - Gingival hyperplasia

3
Oral Surgery

3.1   Local anaesthetics

(a) You plan to extract a lower left first permanent molar tooth on a fit
and healthy 34-year-old patient using 25% lidocaine with adrenaline
1:80 000. You plan to carry out an inferior dental/alveolar block,
but what other nerves will you need to anaesthetise for the
extraction to be carried out, and which injections will you give to
achieve this?

(b) Once you have given your injections how will you test each nerve to
see whether it is anaesthetised?

(c) What are the techniques for giving an inferior dental/alveolar block?
Please give an advantage and disadvantage for each of the
techniques.

(d) The patient is still feeling discomfort when you try to elevate the
tooth. What alternative techniques or anaesthetic agents could you
try?

Answer 3.1

(a) An inferior dental (alveolar) block (IDB) of the nerves will anaesthetise the pulp of the tooth to be extracted. Which technique is used (see section c) for an IDB will determine whether you need to use other injection techniques, eg with certain high IDBs the long buccal nerve is blocked at the same time as the inferior dental/alveolar nerve. Hence, if not already anaesthetised, the long buccal nerve will need to be anaesthetised, because this supplies the buccal tissues adjacent to the tooth.

You will also need to anaesthetise the lingual nerve because this supplies the lingual tissues adjacent to the tooth, and can be given at the same time as the IDB.

(b) To test that the various injection techniques have been successful, you will need to probe in different areas. Probing in the buccal gingival sulcus of the lower first permanent molar to be extracted will test whether the long buccal nerve has been anaesthetised. Probing in the lingual gingival sulcus of the lower first permanent molar to be extracted will test whether the lingual nerve has been anaesthetised. Hence it is necessary to probe at another site to determine whether your IDB has been successful. As the buccal mucosa anterior to the mental foramen will be anaesthetised in a successful IDB, this area can be probed to determine whether the inferior dental/alveolar nerve has been successfully anaesthetised. However, care must be taken not to do this too close to the midine, because there is crossover supply from fibres on the contralateral side and a false-negative result may occur.

(c) IDB techniques are shown below.

Technique of IDB	Advantages	Disadvantages
Direct technique, also known as Halstead's technique	Simple	If needle inserted in wrong position, may encounter internal oblique ridge and prevent advancement to lingula
Indirect technique	Gets round the problem of hitting the internal oblique ridge on insertion of the needle	More movement of needle within tissues
Anterior ramus technique	Can be done in patients with limited mouth opening	Needle movement in the tissues
Gow—Gates technique	Blocks the long buccal nerve at same time, as well as accessory nerve supplies such as the mylohyoid and auricular temporal nerves	Takes longer to work because the nerve trunk is larger at this point Possibility of intravascular injection into maxillary or middle meningeal arteries or veins
Akinosi technique	Can be done in patients with limited mouth opening Blocks long buccal nerve at same time, as well as accessory nerve supplies such as the mylohyoid and auricular temporal nerves	Takes longer to work because the nerve trunk is larger at this point Possibility of intravascular injection into maxillary or middle meningeal arteries or veins

(d) Other techniques that could be used:
- Intraligamentous injection
- Intraosseous injection

Other agents: lidocaine is the gold standard dental local anaesthetic, but in refractory cases it is possible to use articaine as an alternative/adjunctive anaesthetic agent. As a 4% solution, it is stronger than lidocaine and often helps anaesthesia to be achieved in difficult cases.

3.2 (a) You are seeing a patient who needs to have a tooth surgically removed in your practice. One of the principles of flap design is that vital structures should be avoided. Name two vital structures that you should avoid when carrying out surgical tooth removal in the maxilla and the mandible.

(b) What are the other principles to which you should adhere when designing a mucoperiosteal flap for surgical tooth extraction?

(c) You wish to remove a lower left, second premolar tooth; a diagram of the tooth to be removed is shown. Please draw on it where you would place your incisions and explain your reasons for siting them there.

(d) After the procedure you wish to suture the wound. What functions do sutures perform?

(e) Name two different sutures that could be used to suture an intraoral wound and an advantage of each.

Answer 3.2

(a)

- Maxilla: greater palatine artery; nasopalatine nerves and arteries

- Mandible: lingual nerve and mental nerve

(b) Mucoperisoteal flaps that are raised when surgically removing a tooth need to:

- Provide adequate access to the surgical site

- Retain a good blood supply to the mucoperiosteal flap, so the base must be broader than the apex, unless the flap includes a decent-sized artery within the flap

- Avoid vital structures such as local nerves and blood vessels

- Have their margins placed on sound bone and not over the area where you are removing bone

- Be able to be extended if necessary

- Be able to be closed appropriately at the end of the operation

(c) There is no single universally accepted flap design. However, so long as the principles of flap design are adhered to, then the design will be appropriate.

When designing a flap in this area two- or three-sided flaps are appropriate and, depending on preference, some operators will place the relieving incision in a two-sided flap mesially, whereas others will place it distally. It is important to include the whole interdental papilla in the flap to make suturing at the end easier. The relieving incisions must be flared to ensure a larger base than apex for a good blood supply. In the figure are two designs: one a three-sided flap and the other a two-sided flap with a mesial relieving incision.

(d) Sutures primarily approximate and hold the wound margins in the appropriate place to enable them to heal. The smaller the space between the two wound margins, the quicker the wound will heal. Sutures will help in holding the mucoperiosteal flap over bone, which will reduce the risk of it becoming non-vital. Sutures also help haemostasis.

(e)

- *Non-resorbable*:
  - braided: black silk — soft and easy to knot
  - monofilament: Prolene — hygienic
- *Resorbable*:
  - braided: polyglactin (Vicryl) or Polysorb, which is a glycolide/lactide co-polymer — soft, easy to knot, resorbs so patient does not need to have sutures removed
  - monofilament: poliglecaprone 25 (Monocryl) — hygienic, resorbable but slow resorption

3.3 (a) A fit and healthy patient presents to your surgery complaining of recurrent episodes of pain and swelling of the gum in the region of an impacted, lower right wisdom tooth. What is the most likely diagnosis?

(b) A radiograph of the tooth involved is shown here. How would you describe the position of the tooth?

(c) What is the relationship of the inferior dental canal to the tooth, as judged by this radiographic view? What are the likely implications of this appearance and how would you proceed?

(d) Coronectomy: what is the rationale behind a coronectomy and what are the complications of carrying it out?

Answer 3.3

(a) Recurrent pericoronitis

(b) Mesioangularly impacted and partially erupted

(c) The inferior dental canal crosses the root of the tooth and there is a radiolucent band across the root in this area. There is also loss of the superior cortical outline of the inferior dental canal as it crosses the tooth.

This is likely to represent an intimate relationship between the inferior dental nerve and the roots of the tooth, which means that, if the tooth were to be removed, the patient would be at higher risk of damage to the inferior dental canal.

In an ideal world a cone-beam CT (CBCT) scan would be the next step because this would provide a three-dimensional view of the area and provide a definitive answer as to the true relationship between the root and the nerve. If there is an intimate association or if no CBCT scan is available, then to minimise damage to the nerve the treatment options are:

- To leave the tooth *in situ* and treat each episode of pericoronitis as and when it occurs

- To remove the tooth in its entirety but accept that it has a higher than average risk of causing damage to the inferior dental nerve

- To carry out a coronectomy

(d) A coronectomy is a procedure in which the crown of the tooth is removed and the vital roots are retained. The rationale is that not touching the roots will limit damage to the inferior dental nerve, and removing the crown will allow the mucosa to be sutured across to the lingual side, closing the wound primarily and thereby preventing any further episodes of pericoronitis.

The possible complications are infection from or migration of the retained root. In some instances the root becomes mobile when the crown is sectioned and removed, and a mobile root cannot be left *in situ* so it is necessary to surgically remove the whole tooth.

3.4 (a) Which patients should be referred to a specialist for urgent assessment according to the 2005 National Institute for Health and Care Excellence (NICE) guidelines on urgent referrals for suspected oral cancer?

(b) As a general dental practitioner, to whom would you refer a patient for management if you suspected that they had a squamous cell carcinoma of the oral cavity?

(c) What treatment modalities are commonly used for treating squamous cell carcinoma of the oral cavity?

(d) What do you understand by the term palliative care?

Answer 3.4

(a) Any patient with:
  - Unexplained red and white patches (including suspected lichen planus) of the oral mucosa that are painful or bleeding or swollen. Note: a non-urgent referral should be made in the absence of these, ie not painful, bleeding or swollen.

  - Unexplained ulceration of the oral mucosa persisting for more than 3 weeks

  Any adult patient with
  - Unexplained tooth mobility persisting for more than 3 weeks

  - An unexplained lump in the neck which has recently appeared or a lump which has not been diagnosed before that has changed over a period of 3—6 weeks

(b) An oral and maxillofacial surgery consultant who manages oncology patients within a cancer centre would be the best person to manage the patient as the surgeon is part of a multidisciplinary team that can offer the patient holistic care.

  Oral medicine and oral surgery consultants will see patients referred for suspected squamous cell carcinomas (SCCs), and may arrange for biopsies to be performed but as they are not able to offer the patient definitive surgical treatment. Therefore, it would be ideal for the patient to be referred to the person who would be able to diagnose and manage that lesion from the start.

(c)
  - Surgery

  - Radiotherapy

  - Chemotherapy

  - Combination of any of the above

(d) According to the World Health Organization (2003), 'palliative care is an approach that improves the quality of life of patients and their families facing the problems associated with life-threatening illness, through the prevention and the relief of suffering by means of early identification and impeccable assessment and treatment of pain and other symptoms, physical, psychosocial and spiritual'.

3.5 (a) What are bisphosphonates?

(b) You are a general dental practitioner who has a patient who is about to commence treatment with bisphosphonates. How would you manage them?

(c) You have a patient who has been on oral bisphosphonates for 5 years and requires a dental extraction. Describe how you would manage this patient.

Answer 3.5

(a) Bisphosphonate are pyrophosphate analogues that inhibit resorption of bone. Their proposed mechanism of action includes:
- Reduction of bone turnover
- Inhibition of osteoclast activity

(b) Patients about to commence treatment with bisphosphonates should have been informed of the risk and benefits of the chosen drug by the prescribing physician including the risk of medication-related osteonecrosis of the jaw (MRONJ), which was previously known as bisphosphonate-related osteonecrosis of the jaw (BRONJ). The patient ideally should have a dental assessment prior to commencement of the drugs. This is especially important if the patient is to be given high-dose iv bisphosphonates.
- Patients should be informed of the importance of maintaining a high standard of dental health following treatment with bisphosphonate drugs, and the consequences of not doing so.
- Dental hard and soft tissues must be examined for any disease. Any active infection must be treated before commencement of the treatment.
- Any prosthesis must be carefully examined, as mucosal injury and breakdown is the second most commonly identified risk factor for MRONJ.
- Teeth which are in an acceptable condition but unlikely to be retained in the long term need careful consideration as future exodontia is a risk factor for MRONJ.
- Any teeth of dubious prognosis must also be removed.
- Patients should be advised on oral hygiene and preventive measures to minimise risk of dental disease.
- Patients must be educated about the signs and symptoms of MRONJ and to seek advice if they have concerns.
- Patients must be made dentally fit before commencement of the drug treatment.

(c) Current evidence would suggest that those at serious risk of MRONJ are likely to have been on iv bisphosphonates for more than 12 months or at least 36 months of oral bisphosphonates. Prevention is the best option and it is generally recommended that high-risk procedures, eg extractions, should be avoided and instead root canal treatment should be considered, even when it is not possible to restore the crown of the tooth to a functional form.

There are some variations in the guidelines for exodontia from different countries, eg oral as oppose to parental (iv) bisphosphonates, and thus it is worthwhile checking your up-to-date local guidelines, in particular, Scottish Dental Clinical Effectiveness Programme (www.scottish.dental.org.uk).

The common steps usually followed are:
1 Preoperatively:

   • Rinse with chlorhexidine mouthwash

   • Prophylactic antibiotics (although this is not universally adopted by all clinicians, hence the need to consult with local guidelines)

2 Conservative surgical technique (atraumatic)

3 Primary closure of soft tissue where possible, without stripping periosteum

4 Postoperatively:

   • Chlorhexidine mouthwash for 2 weeks or until mucosa has healed

   • Antibiotics for 5 days (again this is not universally adopted — see above)

5 Keep the patient under review until the socket has healed

Do not attempt further extractions in other sextants of the mouth until the first socket has healed.

3.6 (a) In order to diagnose MRONJ, certain criteria must be met. What are they?

(b) Apart from bisphosphonate drugs, what other types of drugs are associated with MRONJ? Give an example of each type, and list the conditions for which they are prescribed.

(c) In which conditions might a patient be prescribed bisphosphonate medication?

(d) What are the common routes of administration of bisphosphonate medication?

(e) Which patients are most at risk of getting MRONJ?

(f) Name some local risk factors.

Answer 3.6

(a)
- The patient must be taking or have taken anti-resorptive or anti-angiogenic medication.
- The patient must have exposed bone or bone that can be probed through an intraoral or extraoral fistula in the maxillofacial region that has persisted for more than 8 weeks.
- There must not be a history of radiotherapy to the jaws
- There must be no obvious metastatic disease to the jaws (see Ruggiero SL, Dodson TB, Fantasia J, *et al.* American Association of Oral and Maxillofacial Surgeons. *Journal of Oral & Maxillofacial Surgery* 2014; **72**:1938–56)

(b) Bisphosphonates, along with other anti-resorptive medications such as denosumab are associated with MRONJ. The other group of drugs that are implicated is the anti-angiogenesis drugs such as bevacizumab and sunitinib.

(c) Anti-resorptive drugs are taken for:
- Osteoporosis: both prevention and treatment
- Prevention of skeletal fractures in susceptible individuals
- Paget's disease
- Osteogenesis imperfecta
- Metastatic bone disease (usually in connection with breast or prostate carcinoma)
- Bisphosphonates are also used in the management of patients with multiple myeloma, although other anti-resorptives such as denosumab are not
- Anti-angiogenesis drugs are taken for renal cell carcinoma and gastric tumours

(d) Oral and iv.

(e) Patients who have been on high-dose potent medication by an iv route, usually for the management of malignancies.

(f)

- Mandibular extractions
- All dentoalveolar surgery
- Periodontitis, presence of oral abscesses or infection
- Poor oral hygiene
- Denture-related trauma
- Thin mucosal coverage, eg lingual tori

3.7   A fit and healthy 25-year-old patient attends your dental practice with a 2-day history of a painful, loose left mandibular first permanent molar after he was hit in the face with the cricket ball.

(a) What key questions you would ask the patient?

(b) What radiological investigations if any would you carry out after examination?

(c) Following your examination and investigations, you are concerned that the mobile tooth is a result of a fractured mandible. How would you proceed?

(d) If there was a mandibular fracture which radiological view(s) would demonstrate it?

(e) What treatment is likely to be required in this case?

Answer 3.7

(a) You would take the history and examination as usual to ascertain the current complaint, the history of the complaint, the patient's medical, dental and social history. However, in this type of injury, in particular, you would also want to know:

- The circumstances surrounding the incident

- Any loss of consciousness or any other injuries

- If his occlusion is deranged

- If there is any altered sensation in the distribution of the inferior alveolar/dental nerve

- The state of the tooth before the incident, eg pain and mobility

(b) A panoramic radiograph to obtain an overview of the dentition and mandible. If there is insufficient detail of the region of the lower left mandibular first molar tooth then a periapical radiograph may be warranted to determine whether there is a fracture in the tooth or to determine the periodontal status of the tooth.

(c) Immediately refer the patient to the nearest oral and maxillofacial surgery department for further assessment and management.

(d)

- A dental panoramic radiograph and another view at another angle, usually a posterior-anterior view of the mandible (PA mandible).

- An alternative would be oblique lateral views of the mandible and PA mandible, but the oblique lateral views are often inferior to a panoramic radiograph.

- Cone-beam computed tomography (CT) or standard CT would also provide good information regarding the fracture but is not indicated in simple fractures due to the higher radiation dose relative to a dental panoramic radiograph and PA mandible.

(e) It is likely that the fracture is displaced as the patient feels movement in the lower left first molar. Hence he requires surgical treatment in the form of open reduction and internal fixation of the fractured mandible. For a body of mandible fracture this is often accessed via an intraoral approach.

3.8 (a) A fit and healthy 10-year-old child fell while playing on his micro-scooter and is brought into your surgery with evidence of injury to his maxillary anterior teeth. Your worry is that the child may have sustained an alveolar or dento-alveolar fracture. What are the differences between these two terms?

(b) What features would lead you to suspect that the child had sustained a dento-alveolar fracture?

(c) What investigations would you carry out and what findings would you expect?

(d) Assuming the child is co-operative and there are no other injuries, how would you manage the dento-alveolar fracture?

(e) What post-treatment instructions would you give the patient and his parents?

Answer 3.8

(a) A fracture of the alveolar process may or may not involve the alveolar socket. A dento-alveolar fracture would involve fracture of the alveolar process and the socket.

(b)

- Teeth related to the fractured dento-alveolar segment are typically all mobile and move as a unit.

- An occlusal change will often be present due to the displacement of the entire segment.

- The teeth of the affected segment are often tender to percussion.

(c)

- Vitality testing of all the involved teeth — this is usually negative.

- Radiographs — usually two views are recommended for identification of fractures. Ideally, these should be at right angles to one another for better identification of fracture lines but in practice the views are usually taken with the X-ray tube head in two different positions. In the anterior region the options would be periapical views and an upper standard occlusal. A panoramic or a cone-beam CT may also be useful. Radiographic findings suggestive of a dento-alveolar fracture may present as:

  - A radiolucent line between the fragments. However, the vertical line of the fracture may be difficult to see as it may run along the periodontal ligament space. The horizontal line may be located apical at the apex or coronal to the apex.

  - An alteration in the outline shape of the root and discontinuity of the periodontal ligament

  - An associated fracture(s) of the roots of the teeth.

(d) After gaining consent you would:

  1 Administer local analgesia

  2 Reposition the displaced segment with digital pressure applied both labially and palatally or with forceps if necessary

  3 Stabilise the fractured segment for 4 weeks with flexible splinting, such as:

    - An acid etch splint with composite with or without a wire

- Orthodontic brackets on the teeth and splinting with a flexible sectional archwire

- Preformed trauma arch bars

(e)

- Soft diet for 1 week

- Explain that good oral hygiene is essential for healing of the tissue and that chlorhexidine mouthwash may be beneficial

- Explain the need for longer-term follow-up, as there is the risk of:

    - Pulp necrosis

    - Ankylosis

    - Resorption associated with infection

    - Bone loss

    - Loss of tooth

Current suggested guidelines for follow-up

- Splint removal and clinical and radiographic control after 4 weeks

- Clinical and radiographic control after 6—8 weeks, 4 months, 6 months, 1 year and yearly for 5 years

For further information, please see www.dentaltraumaguide.org

3.9 (a) What does the term pericoronitis mean? Which teeth are most commonly affected by it?

(b) What are the signs and symptoms of pericoronitis?

(c) How do you treat acute pericoronitis?

Answer 3.9

(a) Pericoronitis means infection of the tissue surrounding the crown of a tooth. The lower third molars are most commonly affected.

(b) Depends on the severity of the infection:
  - Mild — swelling of soft tissue around the crown of the tooth, bad taste, pain
  - Moderate — lymphadenopathy, trismus, extraoral swelling
  - Severe — fever, malaise, spreading infection and abscess formation

(c) Treatment depends on the severity of the infection. Management of mild infection includes:
  - Oral hygiene instructions such as cleaning around the tooth and operculum with chlorhexidine or hot salty water
  - Debridement of the area around the tooth and under the operculum
  - Relief of trauma from opposing tooth — grind cusps or extraction of the tooth
  - Analgesics
  - Antibiotics (metronidazole)

Severe infection may need hospitalisation, intravenous antibiotics, removal of the lower third molar and/or incision and drainage.

3.10 (a) What does the acronym NICE stand for?

(b) NICE guidelines gives specific indications for removal of wisdom teeth. List five such indications.

(c) What features on a radiograph would suggest that a wisdom tooth is associated with the inferior dental nerve?

(d) What specific information must be given to a patient prior to removal of an impacted lower wisdom tooth, which you would not give if you were removing an upper wisdom tooth?

Answer 3.10

(a) National Institute for Health and Care Excellence

(b) Surgical removal of impacted third molars should be limited to patients with evidence of pathology such as (any five of the following):
- Caries
- Non-treatable pulpal and/or periapical pathology
- Cellulitis
- Abscess and osteomyelitis
- Internal and external resorption of the tooth or adjacent tooth
- Fracture of tooth
- Tooth/teeth impeding surgery or reconstructive jaw surgery
- Tooth is within the field of tumour resection

(c) Loss, deviation or narrowing of the 'tramlines' of the inferior dental canal, and a radiolucent band across the root of the tooth.

(d) Information specific to lower wisdom teeth: numbness/tingling or altered sensation of the lower lip, chin and tongue which may be temporary or permanent. This information needs to be given to the patient because of the possibility of damage to the inferior dental nerve or the lingual nerve during the procedure.

3.11 (a) What do you understand by the term meal-time syndrome?

(b) Which gland does it affect most commonly and why?

(c) What investigations would you carry out if it affected this gland?

(d) How would you manage an acute episode?

Answer 3.11

(a) Patients who have an obstruction in a duct of a major salivary gland often complain of pain and swelling in the region of that gland on smelling or eating food and also on anticipation of food.

(b) It most commonly affects the submandibular salivary gland because the saliva produced by this gland is a thick mucus type, and the duct is long and has an upward course with a bend at the hilum.

(c) Investigations:
- Bimanual palpation
- Plain radiography — usually a lower occlusal view although a calculus may be seen on a panoramic radiograph.
- Sialography
- Ultrasound
- Scintiscanning

(d) Management of an acute episode:
- Encourage salivation, eg by massaging the gland
- Hot salty mouth baths
- Consider commencing antibiotics
- Arrange review for definitive treatment when acute symptoms have subsided

3.12 (a) A patient complains of an ulcer on their tongue. Which of the following features of the ulcer would make you suspect that it was malignant:

- Indurated
- Rolled edges
- Healing
- Pain
- Size
- A whole crop of ulcers present
- Present on the tip of the dorsum of the tongue
- Present on the lateral border of the tongue
- Healing

(b) Which groups of people are most likely to have oral malignancies?

- Children/young adults/older adults
- Males/females

(c) What are the risk factors for oral malignancy?

(d) What is the most common malignancy of the oral cavity?

(e) What treatment is available for the most common malignancy of the oral cavity?

Answer 3.12

(a) Features suspicious of malignancy:
- Indurated
- Rolled edges
- Present on the lateral border of the tongue

(b) People most likely to have oral malignancies:
- Older adults
- Males

(c) Risk factors for oral malignancy:
- Smoking
- Alcohol consumption
- Intraoral use of tobacco products such as snuff
- Betel nut/pan chewing

(d) Squamous cell carcinoma

(e) Surgery:
- Excision and primary closure
- Excision and reconstruction

Radiotherapy:
- Surgery and radiotherapy (and/or chemotherapy) combined
- Other modalities
- Photodynamic therapy

3.13 (a)   What does the term 'internal derangement of the temporomandibular joint (TMJ)' mean?

(b)   What might a patient with an internal derangement of their TMJ complain of? Please give the underlying reason for the complaint.

(c)   If the internal derangement was unilateral, to which side would the mandible deviate on opening and why?

(d)   If imaging of the TMJ were required, which type would be ideal?

Answer 3.13

(a) A localised mechanical fault in the joint, which interferes with its smooth action

(b) Patients may complain of:

- Clicking of the joint (displacement of the disc prevents the condyle from moving smoothly and if the disc and condyle 'jump' over each other, this is felt by the patient as a click or pop)

- Locking of the joint (the disc may be displaced and prevent the condyle from moving normally within the fossa, which may have the effect of locking of the jaw)

- Pain in the joint (may be due to the joint itself, and alteration in the synovial fluid has been suggested as a cause for arthropathy; there may also be associated muscle spasm which can cause pain)

(c) The mandible would deviate towards the side of the internal derangement. This is because the mandible is able to carry out the hinge movement normally, hence the mouth opens (usually about 1 cm). Further movement is usually due to translation of the condyle. If there is an obstruction on one side that condyle will not translate and move forward. The other condyle continues to move in a normal manner and the midline moves towards the static condyle, ie the side with the internal derangement.

(d) Magnetic resonance imaging (MRI)

3.14 (a) Which branch of the trigeminal nerve is most frequently affected in trigeminal neuralgia?

(b) In which sex and at what age does this occur more commonly?

(c) If you had a patient with symptoms of trigeminal neuralgia who did not fit into the common demographic group, what other condition might they have?

(d) Give five features of the pain of trigeminal neuralgia.

(e) Name two types of medication that are effective in trigeminal neuralgia.

(f) Trigeminal neuralgia affecting the ID nerve of the mandibular branch of the trigeminal nerve may be treated surgically. What procedures do you know that can be used on the distal (peripheral) aspect of the nerve?

(g) Less commonly neuralgia may affect another cranial nerve and patients may present with pain to their dentist. Which nerve is involved?

Answer 3.14

(a) Mandibular > maxillary > ophthalmic

(b) Female > male, mid to old age

(c) Differential diagnosis:
  - Multiple sclerosis
  - A central lesion

(d) Any five of the following:
  - Paroxysmal
  - Trigger area
  - Does not disturb sleep
  - Excruciating pain
  - Shooting
  - Sharp, electric shock, burning character
  - Short acting

(e) Any two of the following:
  - Carbamazepine
  - Phenytoin
  - Gabapentin
  - Lamotrigine
  - Oxcarbazepine
  - Baclofen

(f)
  - Cryotherapy
  - Alcohol injection
  - Nerve sectioning

All the above procedures are done at the point where the nerve enters the mandible at the lingula.

(g) Glossopharyngeal nerve

3.15 (a) What do you understand by the term 'dry socket?'

(b) Give five factors that would predispose a patient to getting a dry socket?

(c) How soon after the extraction does the pain usually start?

(d) How would you manage a patient with a dry socket?

Answer 3.15

(a) It is the localised osteitis that occurs in a socket following removal of a tooth.

(b) Any five of the following:
- Smoking
- Oral contraceptives
- Difficult extractions
- Mandibular extractions
- Posterior extractions
- Single extractions
- Immunosuppression
- Bony pathology

(c) 2–3 days after the extraction.

(d) Steps in the management of dry socket:
1 Reassurance and explanation

2 Give analgesics

3 Debride the socket with chlorhexidine or warm salty water

4 Gentle pack the socket with a dressing, eg Alvogyl

5 Review if necessary

3.16 (a) What are the common signs and symptoms of each of the following conditions? Choose the most appropriate from the list below. Options may be used either once, or not at all.

1 Undisplaced unilateral fractured mandibular condyle

2 Orbital blow-out fracture

3 Bilateral displaced fractured condyles

4 Le Fort III fracture

5 Fractured zygomatic arch

6 Fractured zygoma

7 Fracture of the angle of the mandible

8 Dislocated mandible

Signs and symptoms:

- Anterior open bite
- Anaesthesia/paraesthesia of the infraorbital nerve
- Anaesthesia/paraesthesia of the inferior orbital nerve
- Limited eye movements especially when trying to look upwards
- Trismus
- Pain on mandibular movements but no occlusal alteration
- Anaesthesia/paraesthesia of the inferior dental nerve
- Anaesthesia/paraesthesia of the facial nerve
- Cerebrospinal fluid (CSF) leak from the nose
- Limited mandibular movement possible, but inability to occlude or open wide. The patient appears to have a class III malocclusion, with hollowing of the TMJ area.

(b) What do you understand by the term orbital blow-out? Which part of the orbit is most likely to fracture and why?

Answer 3.16

(a) 1 Undisplaced unilateral fractured mandibular condyle — pain on mandibular movements but no occlusal alteration

2 Orbital blow out fracture — limited eye movements especially when trying to look upwards

3 Bilateral displaced fractured condyles — anterior open bite

4 Le Fort III fracture — CSF leak from the nose

5 Fractured zygomatic arch — trismus

6 Fractured zygoma — anaesthesia/paraesthesia of the infraorbital nerve

7 Fracture of the angle of the mandible — anaesthesia/paraesthesia of the inferior dental nerve

8 Dislocated mandible — limited mandibular movement possible, but inability to occlude or open wide. The patient appears to have a class III malocclusion, with hollowing of the TMJ area.

(b) Orbital blow-out means that the rim of the orbit is intact but some part of the bony orbital wall has been fractured. Usually the floor or the medial wall fractures as the bone is thinnest in these regions.

3.17 (a) For each of the following conditions select the most appropriate medicine from the list below. Each option may be used either once or not at all:

1 Bell's palsy

2 Atypical/idiopathic facial pain

3 Acute pericoronitis

4 Post-surgical pain relief

5 Angular cheilitis

6 Antibiotic cover for an extraction for a patient with a prosthetic heart valve

7 Prevention of post-surgical bleeding

8 Trigeminal neuralgia

Medicine:

- Ibuprofen 40 mg three times daily for 5 days
- Ibuprofen 400 mg three times daily for 5 days
- Carbamazepine 100–200 mg twice daily
- Prednisolone 0.5 mg/kg/every 12 hours for 5 days
- Aciclovir
- Miconazole gel
- Nortriptyline 10 mg continuing prescription
- Metronidazole 200 mg three times daily for 5 days
- Metronidazole 200 mg four times daily for 5 days
- Tranexamic acid mouthwash three times daily for 5 days
- Amoxicillin 3 g
- No medication indicated

(b) Name four local measures that can be used to control post-surgical bleeding?

Answer 3.17

(a) **1** Bell's palsy — prednisolone 0.5 mg/kg/12 hours for 5 days

   2 Atypical/idiopathic facial pain — nortriptyline 10 mg continuing prescription

   3 Acute pericoronitis — metronidazole 200 mg three times daily for 5 days

   4 Post-surgical pain relief — ibuprofen 400 mg three times daily for 5 days

   5 Angular cheilitis — miconazole gel

   6 No medication indicated

   7 Prevention of post-surgical bleeding — tranexamic acid mouthwash three times daily for 5 days

   8 Trigeminal neuralgia — carbamazepine 100–200 mg twice daily

(b) Any four of the following:
- Apply pressure
- Administer local anaesthetic with vasoconstrictor
- Pack with haemostatic dressing, eg Surgicel
- Suture
- Bone wax
- Biting on a swab soaked with tranexamic acid, tranexamic acid mouthwashes
- Acrylic suck-down splint

3.18 (a) What are the aims of management of a fractured mandible?

(b) What are the stages of managing a fractured mandible that needs active treatment?

(c) The most common mode of treatment of fractures of the mandible nowadays involves the use of mini-bone plates across the fracture site. Why is intermaxillary fixation often done along with this?

(d) Give three complications of a fracture of the mandible.

(e) What term is used to describe a fracture that involves both condyles and the symphyseal region, and what is the characteristic mechanism of injury?

Answer 3.18

(a) Restoration of function and aesthetics

(b) Stages of treatment/management
 • Reduction

 • Fixation

 • Immobilisation

 • Rehabilitation

(c) Intermaxillary fixation is done to re-create the patient's original occlusion whilst the fractured bone ends are fixed together. The IMF also allows extra traction to be applied after the operation if needed.

(d) Any three of the following:
 • Non-union

 • Malunion

 • Infection

 • Malocclusion

 • Nerve damage

(e) Guardsman fracture — it is thought to occur when a patient falls on their chin (traditionally Guardsmen fainting on parade — hence the name) or suffers a blow to their chin.

3.19 (a) What signs and symptoms would make you suspect that you have created an oroantral communication following the extraction of an upper first permanent molar?

(b) If you have created an oroantral communication how would you treat it?

(c) If a root is pushed into the antrum how can a surgeon gain access to remove the root once the socket had healed?

Answer 3.19

(a) Signs and symptoms of an oroantral communication:
  - A visible defect or antral mucosa visible on careful examination of socket

  - Hollow sound when suction used in socket

  - Bone with smooth concave upper surface (with or without antral mucosa on it) between the roots of the extracted tooth

(b) Management of an oroantral communication:
  - Surgical closure of the defect by: approximating the palatal and buccal mucosa, but there is usually inadequate soft tissue; buccal advancement flap alone or with buccal fat pad; or palatal rotation flap

  - Advise the patient not to blow the nose for 10 days

  - Some surgeons prescribe broad-spectrum antibiotics, inhalation and nasal decongestants.

(c) By raising a flap in the buccal sulcus in the region of the upper canine/ premolars and removing bone — known as a Caldwell–Luc procedure.

3.20 (a) Fill in the blanks from the list of options below:

Bell's palsy is paralysis of the .... nerve which results in a facial palsy. It may be caused by a .... infection particularly .... Treatment involves a .... course of ...., as well as ....

1 trigeminal/glossopharyngeal/facial

2 bacterial/protozoal/viral

3 herpes simplex virus/Epstein—Barr virus/bovine spongiform encephalopathy

4 short/intermediate/long

5 amoxicillin/prednisolone/gabapentin

6 augmentin/gentamicin/aciclovir

(b) How would you test the function of the nerve involved in Bell's palsy? Select the correct options from the list below.

- Ask the patient to look upwards and downwards

- Ask the patient to look left to right

- Ask the patient to close their eyes

- Ask the patient to smile

- Ask the patient to stick their tongue out

- Ask the patient to purse their lips

- Ask the patient to wrinkle their forehead

- Shine a light into the patient's eye to assess their pupillary response

- Check if the patient can detect sharp/blunt sensation in various positions all over the skin of their face

(c) Why is it important to recognise this condition early?

Answer 3.20

(a) Bell's palsy is paralysis of the *facial* nerve which results in a facial palsy. It may be caused by a *viral* infection particularly *herpes simplex.* Treatment involves a *short* course of *prednisolone,* as well as *aciclovir.*

(b)
- Ask the patient to close the eyes

- Ask the patient to smile

- Ask the patient to purse the lips

- Ask the patient to wrinkle the forehead

(c) Early treatment may prevent permanent disability and disfigurement.

3.21   What are the risks of undertaking elective extractions in the following patients and how can the risks be minimised?

(a) A patient who underwent radiotherapy for an oral squamous cell cancer last year

(b) A patient who underwent radiotherapy for an oral squamous cell cancer 25 years ago

(c) A patient who has haemophilia A

(d) A patient who is HIV positive

(e) A patient who has a prosthetic heart valve

(f) A patient who had a myocardial infarction 6 weeks ago

Answer 3.21

(a) Patients who have had radiotherapy are at risk of getting osteoradionecrosis after extractions. Therefore prevention has a big role in these patients. However, if an extraction is needed, antibiotics are usually given until the socket has healed; this may mean a course of 4 weeks or more.

(b) The effects of radiotherapy do not decrease with time; they are permanent. Hence this patient should be managed in the same way as the patient in (a).

(c) Such patients have factor VIII deficiency and therefore impaired clotting times. The severity of the condition depends on the level of factor VIII activity. All patients who require an extraction should only be treated in collaboration with their haematologist. Management usually involves preoperative blood tests, followed by transfusion of the missing factor and/or desmopressin (which stimulates factor VIII production). Other agents such as ε-aminocaproic acid (Amicar) and tranexamic acid (Cyklokapron) may be used along with local measures: sutures and packing the socket with a haemostatic agent. They are usually treated as inpatients to allow postoperative monitoring.

(d) In terms of cross-infection control, universal precautions should be used. With regard to the extraction, depending on the patient's CD4:CD8 count they may be more likely to get a postoperative infection. This could mean that you would give antibiotics more readily than to a fit and healthy patient.

(e) Patients who have prosthetic heart valves are usually taking an anticoagulant, often warfarin. If they are, the extraction should be performed only when the international normalised ratio (INR) has been checked and is within the range that the operator is happy with. The socket is usually packed with a haemostatic aid to help with haemostasis. Prior to 2008 antibiotic cover was given to patients with prosthetic heart valves to guard against the theoretical risk of infective endocarditis following invasive dental treatment. However, since the National Institute for Health and Care Excellence (NICE) guidelines on prophylaxis against infective endocarditis were published in 2008, antibiotic cover is no longer administered to patients undergoing dental treatment.

(f)   There are no firm guidelines as to when it is best to carry out elective dental extractions following a myocardial infarction. Timing will depend on the individual patient. For a patient who is stable and well following a recent myocardial infarction, there is no need to delay an elective dental extraction under local anaesthesia. In this instance it may be wise to liaise with the patient's physician.

3.22 (a)   From the list below choose the space(s) or site that infection typically spreads into from the following teeth: maxillary lateral incisor, mandibular third molar, maxillary canine:

- Sublingual
- Palatal area
- Submandibular
- Buccal
- Submasseteric
- Lateral pharyngeal
- Retropharyngeal
- Infraorbital area

(b)   What are the boundaries of the submandibular space?

(c)   What are the principles of management of a patient with a dental infection?

Answer 3.22

(a)

- Maxillary lateral incisor — palatal, buccal
- Mandibular third molar
  - Sublingual
  - Submandibular
  - Submasserteric
  - Lateral pharyngeal
  - Retropharyngeal
- Maxillary canine — infraorbital

(b)

- Laterally: mandible below mylohyoid line
- Medially: mylohyoid muscle
- Inferiorly: deep cervical fascia and overlying platysma and skin

(c) Identification and removal of the cause of the infection. Steps are:
   1 Establish drainage of the abscess (intraoral/extraoral)

   2 Commence appropriate antimicrobial treatment

   3 Assess if there is any predisposing factors for infection, eg immunosuppression, diabetes, steroid therapy

   4 Supportive measures, analgesics, fluids, soft diet, etc.

3.23 (a) What do you understand by the TMN classification system and what is it used for?

(b) If a patient with an intraoral tumour is staged as T2 N1 M0 what does it mean?

(c) What does Mx mean?

(d) Lesions may be treated by using a graft or a flap — what do you understand by these terms?

Answer 3.23

(a) It is a classification system for tumours and the letters stand for:
- T — tumour
- N — nodes
- M — metastases

It is used to stage tumours.

(b) The patient has a tumour 2—4 cm in size, with a single ipsilateral lymph node less than 3 cm in diameter and no metastases. This patient has stage III disease.

(c) Distant metastases cannot be assessed.

(d) A graft is a piece of tissue that is transferred by complete separation and gains a new blood supply by ingrowth of new blood vessels. A flap has its own blood supply. They can be 'pedicled', ie their original blood supply is used, or 'free', ie they have to be 'replumbed' into the blood supply at the recipient site.

4
Oral Medicine

4.1

(a) Describe the features shown on this photograph

(b) What symptoms may the patient experience?

(c) How is this managed?

Answer 4.1

(a) This photograph shows the dorsum of the tongue; there are red patches on the surface of the tongue. The patches are areas of smooth depapillation, giving the tongue a map-like appearance. It is known as geographic tongue or erythema migrans.

(b) The patient may describe a discomfort or burning sensation often in association with spicy or acidic foods. Some cases are asymptomatic. The patients will describe changes in site, size and shape of the lesions.

(c)

- Take a through history and examination. Geographic tongue does not usually require treatment.

- Reassure that the lesion is benign. It is also common. Often this is sufficient.

- Advise the patient to avoid certain foods.

- Occasionally a topical analgesic mouthwash or spray, eg benzydamine hydrochloride (Difflam), is recommended.

4.2 (a) A 50-year-patient presents with a brown lesion on the palatal mucosa. What characteristics would make you think it was a malignant melanoma?

(b) How would you manage this patient?

(c) What is the prognosis for such a lesion?

(d) What else could the lesion be if it is a single brown lesion in the palate?

(e) If the patient had presented with multiple small brown lesions in the mucosa what could have been the cause?

Answer 4.2

(a)

- Position — most common on the palate
- Colour — usually dark brown or black (although it is possible for some to be non-pigmented or red)
- Age — commonest between 40—60 years of age
- Often asymptomatic
- The lesions are often firm and rubbery to touch. They are macular or nodular and may ulcerate
- They may cause an enlarged node(s), may bleed or become sore — although these are often late presentations

(b) If there is a suspicion of malignant melanoma, an urgent incisional biopsy is indicated to gain a tissue diagnosis, so the patient must be referred urgently to a suitable clinician

(c) The prognosis for malignant melanomas is poor; median survival is about 2 years.

(d)

- Amalgam tattoo
- Racial pigmentation
- Idiopathic melanotic macule
- Melanotic naevus

(e)

- Oral melanocytic naevi
- Peutz—Jeghers syndrome
- Oral melanotic macules associated with human immunodeficiency virus (HIV) infection
- Addison's disease

4.3 (a) A 50-year-old woman presents to your surgery complaining of a dry mouth. What are the common causes of dry mouth?

(b) How would you determine the cause of the dry mouth?

(c) What are the dental concerns in such a patient?

Answer 4.3

(a)

- Developmental — aplasia/atresia
- Salivary gland disease — Sjögren syndrome (primary/secondary), sarcoidosis, HIV infection, iatrogenic, drug-induced, radiotherapy, graft versus host
- Psychogenic — oral dysaesthesia/burning mouth syndrome, anxiety and depression
- Dehydration — systemic febrile illness, diarrhoea, diabetes mellitus and insipidus, renal failure
- Alcohol
- Mouth breathing
- Iatrogenic drugs — those with anticholinergic, sympathomimetic or diuretic activity

(b) You would take the usual history from the patient to include the complaint, the history of the present complaint, the medical, dental and social history, and you would also ask specific questions to determine the cause of the dry mouth including:

- When do they feel their mouth is dry?
- What have they done to help the situation? Eg frequent sips of water
- Difficulty eating/talking?
- Sore/burning mouth?
- Altered taste?

Systemic questions:

- Their general health and well-being
- Any relevant medical conditions, eg the above-mentioned autoimmune diseases/diabetes/cancer

Extra-oral examination:

- Look for swelling/enlargement of the salivary glands, in particular the parotid glands
- Angular cheilitis
- Dry cracked lips

Intra-oral examination:

- Lobulated/fissured tongue

- Candida
- Stringy saliva or parchment dry mucosa
- New carious lesions

Investigations:
- History and examination may point to the diagnosis but the following investigations may aid the diagnosis of dry mouth:
  - Salivary flow rate
  - Schirmer/slit-lamp test (Sjögren syndrome)
  - Urinalysis/ blood glucose (diabetes)
  - Antinuclear antibodies (ANAs), SSA (anti-Ro), SSB (anti-La) to exclude Sjögren syndrome and sarcoidosis
  - Rheumatoid factor (Sjögren syndrome)
  - Erythrocyte sedimentation rate (Sjögren syndrome or sarcoid but non-specific marker)
  - Serum Immunoglobulin levels (connective tissue disease but non-specific)
  - Labial gland biopsy (see Question 4.8)

(c)

- Development of new carious lesions. Try to discourage these patients from using sugar-containing chewing gum or acidic sweets to help encourage saliva production.
- Consider fluoride mouthwash.
- Candidal infection may be present and require treatment.

4.4 (a) List four possible aetiological factors for recurrent aphthae.

(b) What types of recurrent aphthae are there? How do you differentiate between the types? (eg size, location, number)

(c) How may recurrent aphthae be treated?

Answer 4.4

(a) Any four of the following:
- Genetic predisposition
- Immunological abnormalities
- Haematological deficiencies
- Stress
- Hormonal changes
- Gastrointestinal disorders
- Infections

(b) Minor aphthae may occur singly or in crops and they affect the non-keratinised and mobile mucosa. They are usually less than 4 mm diameter. Major aphthae usually occur as single ulcers, which may be greater than 1 cm in diameter. The masticatory mucosa and dorsum of tongue are often affected. Herpetiform aphthae usually occur in crops of ulcers which are 1–2 mm in diameter, although they may coalesce to form larger ulcers. They occur on non-keratinised mucosa.

(c) Treatment options:
- Treat underlying systemic disease
- Benzydamine (Difflam) mouthwash
- Corticosteroids (Betnesol mouthwash, Betnesol spray)
- Tetracycline mouthwashes
- Chlorhexidine mouthwash

4.5 (a) What is angular cheilitis (stomatitis)?

(b) How does angular cheilitis differ from actinic cheilitis?

(c) List three predisposing factors for angular cheilitis.

(d) Which organisms commonly cause angular cheilitis?

(e) What medicaments could be used to treat this?

Answer 4.5

(a) Inflammation of the skin and the labial mucous membrane at the commissures of the lips.

(b) Actinic cheilitis is a premalignant condition in which keratosis of the lip is caused by ultraviolet radiation from sunlight.

(c) Any three of the following:
- Wearing dentures and having denture-related stomatitis
- Nutritional deficiencies, eg iron deficiency
- Immunocompromised
- Decreased vertical dimension resulting in infolding of the tissues at the corner of the mouth, allowing the skin to become macerated

(d) *Staphylococcus aureus* and *Candida albicans*

(e) Fusidic acid cream and miconazole gel

4.6 (a) Acute pseudomembranous candidiasis or thrush is a presentation of candidal infection in the mouth. List four other ways in which candidal infections may present to a dentist.

(b) What does acute pseudomembranous candidiasis look like in the mouth?

(c) Smears are often taken from acute pseudomembranous candidiasis. How are these smears treated and what do they show?

(d) Name two azole-type drugs and two other drugs, which are not azoles, that are used to treat candidal infections.

Answer 4.6

(a) Any four of the following:
- Acute atrophic candidiasis
- Chronic atrophic candidiasis
- Chronic erythematous candidiasis
- Chronic hyperplastic candidiasis
- Chronic mucocutaneous candidiasis
- Angular stomatitis (cheilitis)
- Median rhomboid glossitis

(b) Whitish-yellow plaques or flecks cover the mucosa, but they can be wiped off, leaving erythematous mucosa underneath.

(c) Smears are Gram stained and show a tangled mass of Gram-positive fungal hyphae as well as leukocytes and epithelial cells.

(d) Drugs used to treat candidal infections:
- Azoles — any two of: ketoconazole, miconazole, fluconazole, itraconazole
- Others — nystatin, amphotericin

4.7 (a) Name the common types of white patches and what may cause them.

(b) What would you call a white patch that cannot be characterised clinically or pathologically as any other disease and which is not associated with any physical or chemical causative agent except the use of tobacco?

(c) What are the clinical features of the different types of white patch referred to in (b)?

(d) A biopsy is usually done for these lesions. What type(s) of biopsy would be appropriate?

(e) How are these lesions treated?

Answer 4.7

(a) Common white patches and their causes:
- Frictional keratosis — friction

- Leukoedema — a variation of normal

- Candidal infection — *Candida albicans* infection

- Cheek biting — trauma from cheek biting

- Fordyce spots/granules — developmental (sebaceous glands in the mucosa)

- Lichen planus — unknown (lichen planus from graft-versus-host disease is uncommon)

- Lichenoid reactions — gold/antimalarials/dental amalgam

- Skin grafts — previous free flap to transfer tissue to cover an intraoral defect

(b) Leukoplakia

(c) Types of leukoplakia:
- Homogeneous leukoplakias

- Nodular leukoplakias

- Speckled leukoplakias

(d) Incisional and brush biopsies are appropriate

(e) Treatment options for leukoplakia:
- Removal of causative agent (smoking)

- Surgical removal (traditional surgical techniques or with a laser)

- Photodynamic therapy

- Retinoids

- Specialist referral

- Regular review and biopsy as appropriate

4.8 (a) Sjögren syndrome is a well-known cause of a dry mouth. Name four other causes of dry mouth.

(b) What is the difference between primary and secondary Sjögren syndrome?

(c) What type of biopsy is often carried out to diagnose Sjögren syndrome and why?

(d) What microscopic features would the biopsy show if the patient had Sjögren syndrome?

(e) What other investigations could be carried out to diagnose Sjögren syndrome?

Answer 4.8

(a) Any four of the following:
  - Radiotherapy in the region of the salivary glands
  - Diabetes
  - Dehydration
  - Mumps
  - HIV infection
  - Anxiety states
  - Diuretics
  - Sarcoidosis
  - Amyloidosis
  - Drugs (eg antimuscarinics, antihistamines, antidepressants)

(b) Primary Sjögren syndrome comprises dry mouth and dry eyes. In secondary Sjögren syndrome there is dry mouth and dry eyes in association with a connective tissue disease eg rheumatoid arthritis, systemic lupus erythematosus.

(c) Labial salivary gland biopsy. This is because the minor glands are usually involved at a microscopic level even though they may not be enlarged.

(d) Focal collections of lymphoid cells are seen adjacent to blood vessels, and the greater the number of foci the worse the disease. There is also acinar atrophy.

(e) Investigations for Sjögren syndrome:
  - Blood tests — antinuclear antibodies, SSA (anti-Ro), SSB (anti-La); rheumatoid factor; erythrocyte sedimentation rate
  - Parotid salivary flow rate
  - Schirmer's test
  - Sialography

4.9 The following diseases/conditions may have signs and symptoms that are seen in and around the mouth. Match the disease/condition with the oral signs and symptoms.

Acute leukaemia	Moon molars *Syphilis*
AIDS	Fissured tongue *M-R Downs*
Rheumatoid arthritis	Multiple odontogenic keratocystic tumours *Gorlin Goltz*
HIV carrier	Multiple supernumerary teeth *Cleidocranial*
Melkersson—Rosenthal syndrome	Hairy leukoplakia *EBV, HIV*
Peutz—Jeghers syndrome	Perioral pigmentation *Peutz Addisons*
Gorlin—Goltz syndrome	Koplik's spots *Measles*
Crohn's disease	Recently developed anterior open bite *RhA*
Measles	Kaposi's sarcoma *HIV*
Marfan syndrome	Gingival hypertrophy and bleeding *leukaemia*
Syphilis	High-arched palate *Marfan*
Cleidocranial dysostosis	Wickham's striae *Lichen Planus*
Lichen planus	Cobblestoned buccal mucosa *Crohns*

Answer 4.9

Acute leukaemia	Gingival hypertrophy and bleeding
AIDS	Kaposi's sarcoma
Rheumatoid arthritis	Recently developed anterior open bite
HIV carrier	Hairy leukoplakia
Melkersson—Rosenthal syndrome	Fissured tongue
Peutz—Jeghers syndrome	Perioral pigmentation
Gorlin—Goltz syndrome	Multiple odontogenic keratocystic tumours
Crohn's disease	Cobblestoned buccal mucosa
Measles	Koplik's spots
Marfan syndrome	High-arched palate
Syphilis	Moon molars
Cleidocranial dysostosis	Multiple supernumerary teeth
Lichen planus	Wickham's striae

4.10 (a) What do you understand by the term 'erythroplasia?'

(b) What is often seen histologically?

(c) Put the following lesions in order of malignant potential with the most malignant first.

- White sponge naevus

- Erythroplasia

- Leukoplakia

- Speckled leukoplakia

(d) In the following conditions coloured lesions may appear in the mouth. What colour are they and are they localised or generalised?

- Kaposi's sarcoma

- Haemangioma

- Amalgam tattoo

- Addison's disease

- Irradiation mucositis

Answer 4.10

(a) Erythroplasia is any lesion of the oral mucosa that presents as a red velvety plaque, which cannot be characterised clinically or pathologically as any other condition.

(b) The lesions often show dysplasia or even carcinoma *in situ* or frank carcinoma histologically.

(c) Erythroplasia > speckled leukoplakia > leukoplakia > white sponge naevus

(d)

- Kaposi's sarcoma — reddish purplish (localised)
- Haemangioma — red/purple (localised to area of haemangioma)
- Amalgam tattoo — blue/black (localised)
- Addison's disease — brown patches (localised to certain areas, eg occlusal line)
- Irradiation mucositis — red (generalised in region of irradiation)

4.11 (a) A 45-year-old patient presents with a lump in the palate. Give four possible diagnoses.

(b) List four factors in the history that may help with the diagnosis.

(c) Give four clinical features that may help you decide on the diagnosis.

(d) What investigations may be used to aid the diagnosis?

Answer 4.11

(a) Any four of the following:
- Torus palatinus
- Unerupted tooth
- Dental abscess
- Papilloma
- Neoplasm (benign/malignant) — salivary (pleomorphic adenoma/adenocarcinoma); squamous cell carcinoma; lymphoma

(b) Any four of the following:
- Duration of the lump
- Associated features, eg toothache/periodontally involved teeth
- Any change in size/consistency
- Any exacerbating factors, eg loose denture, denture granuloma, trauma
- Any medical conditions which may be associated with the lump, eg neurofibromatosis, drugs, hormonal, other malignancies

(c) Any four of the following:
- Position of the lump (eg in the midline — developmental torus palatinus)
- Consistency (fluid — pus/blood/cystic fluid; soft, firm, hard — tumour; bony hard — tooth, torus palatinus)
- Colour (eg red — vascular lesion or Kaposi's sarcoma)
- Discharge (pus/blood/cystic fluid)
- Surface texture (uniform/nodular or ulcerated may indicated tumour; anemone-like — papilloma)
- Associated features (eg carious upper first molar)

(d) Investigations:
- Imaging (plain radiography: panoramic radiograph, upper standard occlusal, long cone periapical)
- Computed tomography/cone beam CT
- Biopsy (fine-needle aspiration; incisional/punch biopsy; excisional)
- Blood test if suspicion of underlying blood dyscrasia

4.12 (a) List eight features that one needs to determine in a patient presenting with pain.

(b) Which features would make you think a patient had atypical/idiopathic facial pain?

(c) What treatment is there for atypical/idiopathic facial pain?

Answer 4.12

(a) Any eight of the following:
- Type/character of the pain
- Onset
- Duration of each episode
- Periodicity
- Site
- Radiation
- Severity
- Exacerbating and relieving factors
- Associated factors
- Previous treatment
- Effect on sleep

(b) Features of atypical/idiopathic facial pain:
- Pain unrelated to the anatomical divisions of nerves, and often crossing the midline
- No organic cause can be found
- Investigations do not show anything abnormal
- Long-standing and continuous, often with no exacerbating or relieving factors
- Conventional analgesics provide no relief
- Often described as unbearable

(c) Atypical/idiopathic facial pain is usually managed medically. The drugs of choice include tricyclic antidepressants, eg nortriptyline, amitriptyline, doxepin, trazodone, dosulepin, fluoxetine. It may also be managed with cognitive behavioural techniques.

4.13 (a) A 30-year-old man presents with weakness on the left side of his face. Name two possible intracranial and two possible extracranial causes.

(b) How will you tell whether a nerve lesion causing a facial weakness had an upper motor neuron cause or a lower motor neuron cause?

(c) What is Ramsay—Hunt syndrome?

(d) What treatment is indicated?

Answer 4.13

(a) Extracranial — any two of the following:
- Bell's palsy
- Malignant parotid neoplastic
- Post-parotidectomy
- Sarcoidosis (Heerfordt syndrome)
- Incorrect administration of local anaesthetic
- Melkersson–Rosenthal syndrome

Intracranial — any two of the following:
- Cerebrovascular accident (strokes)
- Intracranial tumour
- Multiple sclerosis
- HIV
- Lyme disease
- Ramsey–Hunt syndrome
- Trauma to base of skull

(b) In a lower motor neuron lesion, the patient cannot wrinkle their forehead on the affected side, but in an upper motor neuron lesion they retain movement of their forehead. Hence to determine which one it is, you need to ask the patient to raise the eyebrows and wrinkle the forehead.

(c) Herpes zoster infection of the geniculate ganglion which produces a facial palsy. There will also be vesicles in the region of the external auditory meatus and the palate due to the viral infection.

(d) Aciclovir. A short course of high-dose steroids is also recommended by some although this is not universally accepted.

4.14   Fill in the blanks in this paragraph on herpes zoster. The words in brackets will give you a clue.

Herpes zoster is caused by the .... (organism) which lies latent in .... It tends to affect .... (age) patients. The chief complaint is .... The lesions are in the form of .... The treatment is .... at a dose of .... mg five times a day for .... Medication for pain relief is also prescribed and .... (another drug) may also help with the pain and speed healing. Postherpetic neuralgia is .... and persisting for more than .... months.

Answer 4.14

Herpes zoster is caused by the *varicella-zoster virus* which lies latent in *dorsal root ganglia*. It tends to affect *middle-aged or older* patients. The main complaint is *pain or tenderness in dermatomes*. The lesions are in the form of *rash, vesicles or ulcerations*. The treatment is *systemic aciclovir* at dose of *200—800* mg five times a day for *7 days*. Medication for pain relief is also prescribed and *systemic corticosteroids* may also help with the pain and speed healing. Postherpetic neuralgia is *pain developing during the acute phase of herpes zoster* and persisting for more than *6 months*.

4.15 (a) Give four causes of localised gingival swelling(s).

(b) For the above four causes, which features and/or what additional investigation would aid the diagnosis.

Answer 4.15

(a) Any four of the following:
- Periodontal abscess

- Fibrous epulis

- Denture-induced granuloma

- Pregnancy epulis

- Papilloma

- Giant cell lesion/epulis

- Tumour

(b) See according to what you have chosen from the above list:
- Periodontal abscess — associated with deep periodontal pocket and/ or non-vital tooth

- Fibrous epulis — firm, pink/red may be associated with poor oral hygiene, an excisional biopsy

- Denture-induced granuloma — excisional biopsy and treat the cause, ie poorly fitting denture

- Pregnancy epulis — red lesion associated with pregnancy gingivitis, excised post partum if still present

- Papilloma — white cauliflower-like lesion, excisional biopsy

- Giant cell lesion/epulis — purple—red lesion, radiograph, excisional biopsy and curettage, blood test to exclude central giant cell granuloma and hyperparathyroidism

- Tumour — urgent referral to surgeon for incisional biopsy, radiography to look for bony involvement and CT and magnetic resonance imaging (MRI) to stage the disease

4.16 (a) What are the signs and symptoms of primary herpetic gingivostomatitis?

(b) What is the causative agent?

(c) How would you treat it?

(d) Primary herpetic stomatitis may be followed by recurrent herpes labialis. How does this happen?

(e) Describe the lesions of herpes labialis and how you would manage them.

Answer 4.16

(a) Patients have multiple vesicles in their mouth, which burst to leave painful ulcers. There is often gingivitis. Patients feel generally unwell with fever and malaise. There is cervical lymphadenopathy.

(b) Herpes simplex virus (DNA virus)

(c) Treatment of primary herpetic gingivostomatitis:
- Bed rest, soft diet, fluids, analgesics
- Chlorhexidine or tetracycline mouthwash to prevent secondary infection of the ulcers
- Aciclovir in severe cases or medically compromised patients

(d) The virus remains dormant in the trigeminal ganglion and can be reactivated by factors such as sunlight, stress, menstruation, immunosuppression, common cold or fever.

(e) Lesions appear at the mucocutaneous junction of the lips. The patient often has a prodromal itching/prickling sensation prior to the appearance of the lesion, which starts off as a papule and then forms vesicles that burst leaving a scab. They usually heal without scarring after 7–10 days. The lesions will heal without treatment but if given early, ie in the prodromal phase, antiviral cream such as penciclovir or aciclovir may prevent lesions from occurring or at least speed the healing.

4.17 Select from the list the most appropriate diagnostic test for the various conditions/diseases. Each option may be used only once.

Condition/disease	Diagnostic test
Sjögren syndrome *ESR, Autoantibodies*	Full blood count
Dental abscess causing submandibular space infection	History and clinical examination
Benign mucous membrane pemphigoid	Lower standard occlusal radiograph
Burning mouth	Autoantibody blood tests
Glandular fever	Immunohistochemistry
Giant cell arteritis	Serum angiotensin-converting enzyme
Acute pseudomembranous candidiasis	Erythrocyte sedimentation rate
Sarcoidosis	Paul–Bunnell test
Trigeminal neuralgia	Culture and sensitivity
Submandibular duct salivary calculus	Smear

Answer 4.17

Condition/disease	Diagnostic test
Sjögren syndrome	Autoantibody blood tests
Dental abscess causing submandibular space infection	Culture and sensitivity
Benign mucous membrane pemphigoid	Immunohistochemistry
Burning mouth	Full blood count
Glandular fever	Paul—Bunnell test
Giant cell arteritis	Erythrocyte sedimentation rate
Acute pseudomembranous candidiasis	Smear
Sarcoidosis	Serum angiotensin-converting enzyme
Trigeminal neuralgia	History and clinical examination
Submandibular duct salivary calculus	Lower standard occlusal radiograph

In patients with trigeminal neuralgia, consider requesting MRI of the brain, especially in young patients, because this may be the presenting feature of multiple sclerosis.

4.18 (a) The picture shows the buccal mucosa of a 45-year-old man.
What is the name of this common condition?

Red ς white

(b) This condition may have other presentations in the mouth. Name
four.   *Gingivae , erosions/ulcers, tongue .*

(c) Where else may the patient get lesions in the mouth?

(d) In which extraoral sites may such lesions occur and what are they
like?

(e) This condition may be caused by certain drugs. Name three such
drugs.
      ACE
      Bblockers
      NSAIDS

Answer 4.18

(a) Lichen planus /lichenoid reaction

(b) Any four of the following:
- Reticular (as in the picture on page 249)

- Atrophic

- Desquamative gingivitis

- Erosive

- Papular

- Plaque like

(c) Dorsum of tongue and gingiva

(d) Extraoral sites:
- Flexor surfaces of wrists (purplish, papular, itchy)

- Genitals (similar to oral lesions)

- Nails (ridges)

- Head (alopecia)

(e) Any three of the following:
- β-Blockers

- Oral hypoglycaemics

- NSAIDs (non-steroidal anti-inflammatory drugs)

- Gold

- Penicillamine

- Some tricyclic antidepressants

- Antimalarials

- Thiazide diuretics

- Allopurinol

4.19   Fill in the blanks using words from the list below. Each word can only be used once.

.... disease is due to sensitivity to .... Patients may suffer from malabsorption of ...., ... and ...., and may have the following oral signs: ...., ... and .... disease is a chronic .... that may affect any part of the gastrointestinal tract, but most commonly affects the .... Oral signs may be seen such as mucosal tags, ..., ... and ....

1   crohn's/irritable bowel syndrome/coeliac disease/granulomatous disease/ulcerative colitis

2   gluten/vitamin B$_{12}$/folate/iron/vitamin C/vitamin D

3   cobblestone mucosa/lip swelling/oral ulceration/lichen planus/ angular cheilitis/glossitis/gingival swellings/

4   ileum/jejunum/stomach

Answer 4.19

Coeliac disease is due to sensitivity to *gluten.* Patients may suffer from malabsorption of *vitamin B₁₂, folate* and *iron*, and may have the following oral signs: *oral ulceration, angular cheilitis* and *glossitis. Crohn's* disease is a chronic *granulomatous* disease that may affect any part of the gastrointestinal tract, but most commonly affects the *ileum.* Oral signs may be seen such as mucosal tags, *cobblestone mucosa, lip swelling* and *oral ulceration.*

5

Oral Pathology

5.1 (a) Describe the signs and symptoms of the following viral conditions:

- Primary herpetic gingivostomatitis

- Herpes labialis

- Hand, foot and mouth disease

(b) Which viruses cause the above conditions?

(c) Describe the histopathological features that would be seen if a biopsy of a herpetic lesion were taken. How do these differ from the histopathological features of a vesicle seen in pemphigus vulgaris?

Answer 5.1

(a)

- Primary herpetic gingivostomatitis: dome-shaped vesicles, measuring about 2–3 mm, can occur anywhere within the oral mucosae, but commonly affect the hard palate and dorsum of the tongue. The vesicles then rupture, leaving circular shallow ulcers. There is often gingivitis as well. The regional lymph nodes may also be enlarged, and the patient is often systemically unwell with fever.

- Herpes labialis: this is caused by reactivation of the latent herpes simplex virus, which remains in the trigeminal ganglion and is reactivated by factors such as cold, sunlight, local irritation or menstruation. The patient will get a prodromal sensation of burning or tingling, which is followed by redness at the site of the lesion. Vesicles then appear at the mucocutaneous junction of the lips and sometimes on the nose or skin around the mouth, and then coalesce and weep exudate. The lesions then crust over.

- Hand, foot and mouth disease: patients usually develop ulceration throughout the mouth, and also a vesicular rash on the hands and feet.

(b) The infections are caused by:
- Primary herpetic gingivostomatitis: herpes simplex virus type 1

- Herpes labialis — a herpex simplex virus

- Hand, foot and mouth disease: Coxsackie A virus

(c) Histopathological examination of a herpetic lesion reveals dome-shaped vesicles in the upper layers of the epithelium. At the base of the vesicle, the epithelial cells are damaged by the virus and have swollen nuclei and ballooning degeneration. Multinucleated cells are also seen.

Vesicles of pemphigus vulgaris are also intraepithelial, often starting with clefts that extend to form vesicles. There is separation of the suprabasal spinous cells due to antibodies to desmosomal proteins. The keratinocytes become rounded and the cytoplasm contracts around the nucleus. This loss of keratinocyte cell attachment is known as acantholysis. Groups of the rounded-up cells can often be seen within the vesicle. Ruptured vesicles may also be seen. The base of the vesicle may have lined-up basal cells — a tombstone effect covering the basement membrane.

Immunohistochemistry will detect binding of antibodies to desmoglein 3, a desmosomal protein.

5.2 (a) What are the two types of fibrous dysplasia?

(b) Describe the key clinical features of each type.

(c) Describe the key histopathological features of fibrous dysplasia.

Answer 5.2

(a) Monostotic and polyostotic.

(b) Monostotic fibrous dysplasia:
- This is the commonest fibrous dysplasia; it can affect any bone but if it occurs in the jaws the maxilla is more commonly affected than the mandible.
- Usually affects children or adolescents, but may not be diagnosed until later in life.
- Usually present as a gradual smooth bony swelling
- Fibrous dysplasias are usually painless
- Radiographs may show a variety of appearances, and it is often difficult to tell where the lesions end as there may be a gradual transition to normal bone.
    - The lesions do not tend to cross suture lines.
    - Depending on the stage of the condition the lesions may be radiolucent when they first appear but as time goes on more bony trabeculae appear and the lesions become more mottled and opaque.
    - They are sometimes described as having an orange peel or ground glass appearance.
    - Teeth may be displaced.

Polyostotic fibrous dysplasia:
- Less common than monostotic fibrous dysplasia
- Female:male ratio: 3:1
- Variable distribution of lesions, but may be confined to one segment or side of the body
- Usually diagnosed in childhood as patients tend to experience pathological fractures
- May be part of the McCune—Albright syndrome, which also includes precocious puberty, skin lesions and some endocrine abnormalities

(c)

- Normal bone is replaced by fibrous tissue.
- Fibrous tissue may be cellular or very fibrous containing collagen fibres.
- Immature woven bone within islands in the fibrous tissue, which has the appearance of Chinese characters as it is delicate in appearance and irregular in shape.
- The affected bone fuses with normal bone at the margins of the lesions.
- As the lesions mature, woven bone is replaced with lamellar bone.

5.3 (a) Which of the following are histopathological features of epithelial dysplasia?

- Drop-shaped rete ridges
- Nuclear hypochromatism
- Decreased mitotic activity
- Loss of intercellular adherence
- Loss of differentiation
- Saw-tooth rete ridges
- Nuclear pleomorphism
- Civatte bodies
- Loss of polarity of cells

(b) What is the difference between epithelial dysplasia, carcinoma *in situ* and carcinoma?

(c) What is the commonest cancer of the oral cavity?

(d) Give three risk factors for this oral cancer.

(e) If a patient has a suspicious looking ulcer on the lateral border of their tongue what type of biopsy would be carried out to aid diagnosis and why, and what should be included in the biopsy?

Answer 5.3

(a) Histopathological features of epithelial dysplasia:
- Drop shaped rete ridges
- Loss of intercellular adherence
- Loss of differentiation
- Nuclear pleomorphism

(b) Epithelial dysplasia is usually graded histologically as mild, moderate and severe. The term carcinoma *in situ* is often used to describe severe dysplasia in which the changes are seen in all the layers of the epithelium. However, the changes are confined to the epithelium in dysplasia and carcinoma *in situ*, whereas in carcinoma the changes are seen to extend through the basement membrane into the underlying connective tissue.

(c) Squamous cell carcinoma

(d) Any three of the following:
- Alcohol
- Tobacco
- Betel nut chewing
- Human papilloma virus
- Syphilis
- Chronic candidal infection

(e) Incisional biopsy. This should include some normal surrounding tissue and a representative portion of the lesion. Incisional biopsies are preferred so that some of the lesion is left to aid the surgeon (who may not have performed the biopsy) should they need to completely remove the lesion at a later date.

5.4 (a) From the options below select the correct descriptions of giant cell granulomas

- They occur most commonly in the first to third decades/fourth to fifth decades/sixth decade plus.

- They are more common in males than females/females than males.

- They affect the maxilla/mandible most commonly.

- They occur anteriorly/posteriorly most commonly.

(b) Name three pathological features that you might see in a giant cell granuloma.

(c) Why would you do blood tests for a patient with a giant cell granuloma?

(d) What two blood tests would you do and why?

(e) Name two other non-odontogenic benign tumours of bone that affect the jaws.

Answer 5.4

(a) Regarding giant cell granulomas:
- They occur most commonly in the *first to third decades.*
- They are more common in *females than males.*
- They affect the *mandible* most commonly.
- They occur *anteriorly* most commonly.

(b) Any three of the following:
- Giant cells (osteoclasts)
- Vascular stroma/connective tissue
- Spindle-shaped cells
- Haemosiderin (evidence of bleeding)
- Fibroblasts and evidence of collagen formation
- Osteoid

(c) Pathologically giant cell granulomas are identical to brown tumours of hyperparathyroidism. Blood tests help to distinguish between the two conditions. The blood chemistry is normal in giant cell granuloma but altered in hyperparathyroidism.

(d) Any two of the following:
- Plasma calcium levels — raised in hyperparathyroidism, normal in giant cell granuloma
- Alkaline phosphatase levels — lowered in hyperparathyroidism, normal in giant cell granuloma
- Plasma phosphate levels — lowered in hyperparathyroidism, normal in giant cell granuloma
- Parathyroid hormone levels — raised in hyperparathyroidism, normal in giant cell granuloma

(e) Any two of the following:
- Osteoma
- Osteochondroma
- Melanotic neuroectodermal tumour

5.5 (a) What is the definition of a cyst?

(b) Are the following lesions inflammatory/developmental/non-epithelial/neoplastic:

- Keratocystic odontogenic tumours (odontogenic keratocysts)
- Dentigerous cysts
- Radicular cysts
- Aneurysmal bone cyst

(c) From what are dentigerous cysts thought to arise and why?

(d) Where do dentigerous cysts occur most commonly?

(e) Describe what the lining and capsule of a dentigerous cyst would look like histologically.

Answer 5.5

(a) A cyst is a pathological cavity, not formed by the accumulation of pus, with fluid, semifluid or gaseous contents, and lined by epithelium.

(b) Type of lesion:
   - Keratocystic odontogenic tumours (odontogenic keratocyst) — developmental/neoplastic

   - Dentigerous cysts — developmental

   - Radicular cysts — inflammatory

   - Aneurysmal bone cyst — non-epithelial

   According to the World Health Organization (WHO) classification (2005) keratocystic odontogenic tumours are now classified as neoplastic, whereas previously they were thought to be developmental.

(c) Dentigerous cysts are attached to an unerupted tooth in the region of the amelocemental junction and so are thought to arise from the remnants of the enamel organ. The internal enamel epithelium lies over the enamel and the external enamel epithelium forms the cyst lining.

(d) They are associated with teeth that fail to erupt and so are most commonly associated with mandibular third molars and maxillary permanent canines.

(e) The lining is a thin regular layer composed of stratified squamous epithelium, which may occasionally keratinise. The capsule is composed of collagenous fibrous tissue, which is usually free from inflammatory cells. There may be scattered nests of quiescent odontogenic epithelium

5.6 (a) What is the difference between a potentially malignant (premalignant/epithelial precursor) lesion and a potentially malignant (premalignant) condition?

(b) What do you understand by the term leukoplakia?

(c) Put the following lesions in order with the one most likely to become malignant first:

- Leukoplakia

- Speckled leukoplakia

- Erythroplasia (erythroplakia)

(d) What malignancy would they turn into?

(e) At which intraoral sites does oral cancer occur commonly?

(f) How does this cancer spread?

(g) What factors would affect survival from oral cancer?

Answer 5.6

(a) A premalignant lesion is a lesion in which carcinoma may develop. A premalignant condition is a condition in which there is a risk of carcinoma developing within the mouth, but not necessarily in the pre-existing lesion.

(b) A white patch or plaque that cannot be characterised clinically or pathologically as any other disease and is not associated with any physical or chemical agent except the use of tobacco. It cannot be rubbed off.

(c) Erythroplasia (erythroplakia) > speckled leukoplakia > leukoplakia

(d) Squamous cell carcinoma

(e) Common sites of oral cancer:
- Lateral border of tongue
- Floor of mouth
- Retromolar area

(f) Modes of spread:
- Direct extension into adjacent tissues
- Metastasis to regional lymph nodes
- Late in the disease there may be haematogenous spread

(g)
- Delay in treatment
- Size of tumour at presentation
- Degree of differentiation of tumour — poorly differentiated worse than well differentiated
- Lymph node spread
- Distant metastases
- Position of tumour — more posterior worse prognosis
- Malnutrition
- Age, worse with advancing age
- Males have a worse prognosis compared with females

5.7 (a) In which gland do salivary calculi occur most commonly and why?

(b) What symptoms might a patient with a salivary gland obstruction complain of?

(c) Are calculi a common cause of dry mouth?

(d) If a salivary calculus is not treated what may happen to the gland and what would it look like histologically?

(e) What do you understand by the term mucocele. What are the types of mucocele and how do they differ?

Answer 5.7

(a) Submandibular salivary gland. This is because of the composition of saliva produced by this gland, and the length and anatomy of the duct.

(b) Meal time syndrome — they complain of pain and swelling in the region of the gland on seeing, smelling or tasting food. The swelling gradually subsides over time. The gland may also become infected.

(c) No

(d) The gland may become infected and the patient may develop chronic sialadenitis. There is dilatation of the ductal system, and hyperplasia of the ductal epithelium and development of squamous metaplasia. There is destruction of the acini which are replaced by fibrous tissue. Histologically, there is chronic inflammatory cell infiltration of glandular parenchyma.

(e) A mucocele is a cyst of a salivary gland, which commonly forms in the lower lip. They can be *extravasation cysts* where the saliva leaks into the surrounding tissues forming a *cyst-like space* without an epithelial lining. Much less common are *retention cysts*, where the saliva remains within the ductal system and the duct dilates to form a cyst, which is lined by epithelium. A *ranula* is a mucocoele which arises in the floor of the mouth from the sublingual salivary gland or the submandibular gland.

5.8 Fill in the blanks using words from the following lists.

(a) Cherubism is inherited as an .... It usually affects ....
Bilateral bony swellings are seen in the .... and the
.... Histologically the lesions consist of .... in
vascular ....

1 sex-linked trait/autosomal recessive trait/autosomal dominant trait

2 young children/young adults/middle aged

3 tuberosities/frontal region/maxillae

4 angles of the mandible/body of the mandible/symphysis of the
mandible

5 giant cells/Birbeck granules/Civatte bodies

6 connective tissue/epithelium

(b) Primary hyperparathyroidism is caused by .... or adenoma of
the .... This results in .... of parathormone, which in
turn .... the plasma .... level by mobilising calcium.
.... swellings of the jaws can occur. Histologically these
lesions have the characteristics of a .... lesion.

1 hypoplasia/atrophy/hyperplasia

2 pituitary/thyroid/parathyroids

3 over-production/reduction

4 raises/lowers/depletes

5 calcitonin/calcium/vitamin D

6 fibrous/cyst-like/granulomatous

7 tuberculous/granulomatous/giant cell

(c) Paget's disease commonly affects the.................... . Bone resorption
and .... are irregular and exaggerated. This can lead to
.... the foramina and cranial nerve compression. Teeth may
show .... and are often difficult to extract.

1 young/middle-aged/elderly people

2 resorption/replacement/reduction

3 widening of/narrowing of/compression of

4 caries/external resorption/hypercementosis

(d) Osteogenesis imperfecta is also known as .... It is usually
inherited as a(an) .... condition. It is due to defective
synthesis of type .... collagen. Patients may have....................
sclera. Bones grow to .... length, but can be distorted by
multiple fractures and result in dwarfism.

1 brittle bone/marble bone

2 autosomal dominant/autosomal recessive/X-linked

3 I/II/III/IV

4 red/yellow/blue/grey

5 normal/reduced

Answer 5.8

(a) Cherubism is inherited as an *autosomal dominant trait*. It usually affects *young children*. Bilateral bony swellings are seen in the *maxillae* and at the *angles of the mandible*. Histologically the lesions consist of *giant cells* in vascular *connective tissue*.

(b) Primary hyperparathyroidism is caused by *hyperplasia* or adenoma of the *parathyroids*. This results in *over-production* of parathormone, which in turn *raises* the plasma *calcium* level by mobilising calcium. *Cyst-like* swellings of the jaws can occur. Histologically these lesions have the characteristics of a *giant cell* lesion.

(c) Paget's disease commonly affects *elderly people*. Bone resorption and *replacement* are irregular and exaggerated. This can lead to *narrowing of* the foramina and cranial nerve compression. Teeth may show *hypercementosis* and are often difficult to extract.

(d) Osteogenesis imperfecta is also known as *brittle bone* disease. It is usually inherited as an *autosomal dominant* condition. It is due to defective synthesis of *type I* collagen. Patients may have *blue* sclera. Bones grow to *normal* length, but can be distorted by multiple fractures and result in dwarfism.

5.9 (a) What do you understand by the term Nikolsky's sign?

(b) Pemphigus vulgaris and mucous membrane pemphigoid are both blistering diseases, which exhibit this sign. At what level do the blisters occur in the two conditions?

(c) Why do they occur at this level?

(d) Immunohistochemistry is often used to diagnose these conditions. What do you understand by this term? What types are there and how do they differ?

(e) Molecular biology has a role in pathological diagnosis. Name one molecular biological technique.

Answer 5.9

(a) Nikolsky's sign is when a vesicle appears on gently stroking the mucosa or skin.

(b) In pemphigus vulgaris the blisters are intraepithelial. In mucous membrane pemphigoid they are subepithelial.

(c) The two diseases are autoimmune conditions in which autoantibodies are produced against components of the squamous epithelium of the mucosa (and skin). In pemphigus vulgaris autoantibodies are produced against an intercellular adhesion molecule (desmoglein). This causes the keratinocytes to lose their attachment to each other and vesicles/bullae are formed within the epithelium. In mucous membrane pemphigoid autoantibodies are produced against a component of the basement membrane which results in subepithelial separation.

(d) Immunohistochemistry is a technique in which specific antigens within tissue can be visualised with a light or fluorescent microscope. An antibody is applied to a section of tissue and allowed to bind. The binding site is then visualised by a fluorescent 'tag', by means of more antibodies attaching to fluorescent tags or by means of a chemical reaction to produce a colour change. There are two types of immunohistochemistry:
- Direct immunohistochemistry — a section of the patient's tissue is placed on a slide and an antibody against the test antigen is added and allowed to bind. The binding site is then visualised by one of the means described above.

- Indirect — a section of normal tissue (not from the patient) is placed on a slide and serum from the patient is added and allowed to bind. An antibody against the suspected autoantibody in the patient's serum is allowed to bind. The binding site is then visualised by one of the means described above.

(e) Any one of the following:
- Polymerase chain reaction (PCR)

- *In situ* hybridisation

- Northern/Southern/western blotting

5.10   From the right column of the table below select the histopathological features or terms that you would expect to see in the conditions or diagnoses given in the left column. Each condition or diagnosis may have one or more than one histopathological feature.

Conditions/diagnosis	Histopathological features
Lichen planus	Cholesterol clefts
Radicular cysts	Saw-tooth rete ridges
Herpes simplex infection	Ballooning degeneration
Pemphigus vulgaris	Acantholysis
Adenoid cystic carcinoma	Perineural invasion
Denture-induced stomatitis	Acanthosis
White sponge naevus	Rushton's bodies
	Gram-positive hyphae
	Civatte bodies
	Epithelial hyperplasia with basket-weave appearance

Answer 5.10

Conditions/diagnosis	Histopathological features
Lichen planus	Saw-tooth rete ridges, Civatte bodies, acanthosis
Radicular cysts	Cholesterol clefts, Rushton's bodies
Herpes simplex infection	Ballooning degeneration
Pemphigus vulgaris	Acantholysis
Adenoid cystic carcinoma	Perineural invasion
Denture-induced stomatitis	Acanthosis, Gram-positive hyphae
White sponge naevus	Epithelial hyperplasia with basket-weave appearance

5.11   From the right column of the table below select the site where the lesions given in the left column are most likely to occur. Each option may only be used once.

Lesion	Site
Squamous cell carcinoma *Latr*	Palate
Ranula *Fom*	Upper lip
Ameloblastoma *Angle*	Lower lip
Kaposi's sarcoma *Palate*	Dorsum of tongue
Basal cell carcinoma *Skin*	Lateral border of tongue
Mucus extravasation cyst *Lir*	Angle of mandible
Erythema migrans *Porjun*	Parotid gland
Pleomorphic adenoma *Parotid*	Skin of the face
Lichen planus of the skin ———	Flexor surfaces of the wrists
	Floor of mouth

Answer 5.11

Lesion	Site
Squamous cell carcinoma	Lateral border of the tongue
Ranula	Floor of the mouth
Ameloblastoma	Angle of the mandible
Kaposi's sarcoma	Palate
Basal cell carcinoma	Skin of the face
Mucus extravasation cyst	Lower lip
Erythema migrans	Dorsum of the tongue
Pleomorphic adenoma	Parotid gland
Lichen planus of the skin	Flexor surfaces of the wrists

5.12 (a) Please select the most appropriate term/word to fill in the blanks:

Most salivary gland tumours occur in the.................... gland. Most salivary gland tumours in the parotid gland are .... Salivary gland tumours in the .... gland are malignant more often than those in the submandibular gland. Most salivary tumours in the sublingual gland are

....

1 parotid/sublingual/submandibular

2 benign/malignant

(b) Name one benign salivary gland tumour and three malignant salivary gland tumours.

(c) Which salivary gland tumours tend to infiltrate along nerve sheaths?

(d) What do you understand by the term necrotising sialometaplasia?

(e) Where are you likely to see this condition?

(f) What factors predispose to this condition?

Answer 5.12

(a) Most salivary gland tumours occur in the *parotid* gland. Most salivary gland tumours in the parotid gland are *benign*. Salivary gland tumours in the *sublingual* gland are malignant more often than those in the submandibular gland. Most salivary tumours in the sublingual gland are *malignant*.

Note: percentage of malignant tumours: in the parotid glands — 15—32%; in the submandibular glands — 41—44%; in the sublingual glands — 70—90%; and in the minor salivary glands — 50% (WHO 2005).

(b) Benign — any one of the following:
- Pleomorphic adenoma

- Warthin tumour

Malignant — any three of the following:
- Adenoid cystic carcinoma

- Mucoepidermoid carcinoma

- Acinic cell carcinoma

- Carcinoma in ex-pleomorphic adenoma

(c) Adenoid cystic carcinoma and polymorphous low-grade adenocarcinoma

(d) This lesion looks clinically and histologically like a squamous cell or mucoepidermoid carcinoma but is caused by chronic inflammation of minor salivary glands often with necrosis of acini. There is squamous metaplasia of duct tissue.

(e) The palate

(f) Predisposing factors:
- Smoking

- Male

- Middle age

5.13 (a) From which structure are keratocystic odontogenic (odontegenic keratocysts) tumours thought to arise?

(b) Why do keratocystic odontogenic tumours (odontogenic keratocysts) have a strong tendency to recur after removal?

(c) Which age group do they most commonly occur in?

(d) Which is the most common site of presentation?

(e) List four characteristic histological features of odontogenic keratocystic tumours.

(f) What syndrome are odontogenic keratocystic tumours associated with?

(g) What are the characteristic facial features in patients with this syndrome?

(h) What other lesions do these patients present within the head and neck?

Answer 5.13

(a) Dental lamina or its remnants

(b) Reasons for recurrence:
- They are difficult to remove intact due to the thin fragile cyst lining.
- They often have 'daughter' cysts.
- They are multilocular with finger-like extensions within the bone.
- The keratocyst epithelium proliferates rapidly.
- The remnants of the dental lamina may produce more lesions.

(c) 20–30 years

(d) Angle of the mandible

(e) Any four of the following:
- Uniform thickness of epithelium
- Flat basement membrane, 5–10 cells thick
- Elongated palisaded basal cells
- Eosinophilic layer of prekeratin in parakeratinised cyst
- Orthokeratin formation and well defined granular cell layer in orthokeratinised cysts
- Folded cyst lining
- Thin fibrous wall

(f) Basal cell naevus syndrome, Gorlin–Goltz syndrome

(g) Frontal and parietal bossing, broad nasal root

(h) Multiple naevoid basal cell carcinomas

5.14 (a) Lichen planus is a chronic inflammatory disease. Which tissues does it commonly affect?

(b) Which age group is commonly affected?

(c) Reticular lichen planus and atrophic lichen planus are common clinical presentations. Name two other clinical appearances of lichen planus.

(d) List four typical histological features of (reticular) lichen planus

(e) What other histological changes might be seen in the epithelium if the lesion were atrophic?

(f) What serious complication can arise in lichen planus?

(g) Name another connective tissue disorder that can give rise to intraoral lesions similar to lichen planus.

Answer 5.14

(a) Skin and mucous membranes

(b) Over 40 years

(c) Any two of the following:
- Desquamative gingivitis
- Erosive
- Papular
- Plaque like

(d) Any four of the following:
- Hyperkeratosis/parakeratosis
- Saw-tooth rete ridges
- Band-like lymphoplasmacytic infiltration in the juxta-epithelial lamina propria
- Oedema extending into the basal layers resulting in liquefaction degeneration of the basal cell layer
- Lymphocyte infiltration into the basal layers of the epithelium and CD8 lymphocytes predominate
- Hyaline or Civatte bodies in epithelium

(e) There is thinning and flattening of the epithelium

(f) Malignant change

(g) Lupus erythematosus

6
Oral Radiography/ Radiology

6.1   (a)   What do you understand by the terms 'stochastic' and 'deterministic' in relation to radiation damage?

(b)   Radiation dose can be subdivided into three different terms: absorbed dose, equivalent dose and effective dose. What do you understand by each of these terms?

(c)   What factors can influence the effective dose that the patient receives?

Answer 6.1

(a) Stochastic means by chance and so there is no safe radiation dose, because with any dose there is a chance that damage will occur, hence the need to limit exposure wherever possible. Stochastic effects can be divided into somatic effects, where the effects are seen in the individual receiving the radiation, and genetic effects, where the offspring of the individual or future generations are affected.

Deterministic effects are related to dose; they occur only when a threshold dose has been reached and are somatic.

(b)

- Absorbed dose: the mean energy imparted to a unit mass of tissue by ionising radiation. It is measured in grays (Gy) (which are joules per kilogram or J/kg).

- Equivalent dose takes into account the fact that different types of ionising radiation are more damaging to certain types of tissues, so different weightings are given to the absorbed dose. Within dental radiography the absorbed dose and the equivalent dose are the same. It is measured in joules per kilogram but is termed 'sieverts' or Sv.

- Effective dose takes into account the fact that some tissues are more susceptible to the effects of ionising radiation than others. Recent published tissue weightings by the International Commission on Radiological Protection (ICRP) have included the salivary glands, which are an individual weighted tissue and also include oral mucosa. This means that effective doses for dental exposures using the current ICRP weightings are much higher than those used previously.

(c) The effective dose delivered is determined by various factors:
- The sensitivity of the image receptor

- The area exposed to the primary beam

- Exposure factors such as low dose

6.2   What features on a radiograph would make you suspicious of a
malignant process and why?

Answer 6.2

There are certain features that need to be considered when reviewing a lesion on a radiograph. These features, together with the patient's clinical details, eg speed of onset of the lesion or symptom, along with the patient's ethnicity and risk factors, eg smoking, alcohol, known malignant disease elsewhere, are important.

On reviewing a radiograph the following features need to be considered:
- Site
- Size
- Shape
- Outline/poorly defined edge
- Relative radiolucency within the lesion
- Effect on adjacent structure
- Time present

The following features would raise concern:
- Site
- Size
- Shape: irregular shape suggestive of irregular growth, which may indicate a lesion exhibiting destructive growth (eg malignancy) or an inflammatory lesion. Be aware that a solitary bone cyst that is benign typically arches between the roots of teeth.
- Outline/edge or periphery: non-discrete or poorly defined. Rapidly growly lesions such as malignancies are more likely to have non-discrete or poorly defined edge or periphery to a lesion. However, a benign cyst, which usually has a well-defined corticated outline, can become less well defined or even obliterated when it becomes acutely infected, and hence has a more sinister appearance.
- Relative radiolucency within the lesion
- Effect on adjacent structure:
  - Review the effect on the adjacent, teeth, bone and surrounding tissue.

- Resorption of teeth is a feature seen in longstanding benign but locally aggressive lesions and chronic inflammatory lesions, as well as malignancies.

- Surrounding bone may have a ragged destructive appearance. Sinister lesions tend to cause more damage and destruction due to their faster growth pattern.

  - Time present: knowledge of the duration of the lesion can help determine the nature of the lesion. Slow-growing lesions tend to be benign, whereas fast-growing lesions tend to be more aggressive and therefore more likely to be malignant.

6.3 (a) What are the advantages and disadvantages of the various radiographic views you could take to assess the periodontal status of a patient?

(b) When writing a radiographic report regarding periodontal bone loss it used to be common practice to express this in millimetres from the cementoenamel junction (CEJ) to the crest of the alveolar bone. Why is this not considered to be accurate?

(c) What formula is used to represent a more acceptable way to describe the severity of bone loss nowadays?

(d) What are the main patterns of bone loss?

(e) What terms would you use to describe the distribution of bone loss?

Answer 6.3

(a) A dental panoramic radiograph shows the overall degree of bone loss but the detail of the alveolar margin is lost; it also gives a dose of 2.7–3.8 μSv (micro Sieverts) radiation. A horizontal bitewing radiograph will show bone levels in patients with early to moderate disease, but will only show the posterior teeth. Vertical bitewings are useful for teeth with larger probing depths, but again only for posterior teeth. A long-cone periapical radiograph gives the best view as there is minimal distortion and this view can be used for all the teeth in the mouth. They are, however, time-consuming to carry out and give the patient a dose of between 0.3 and 21.6 μSv per periapical film.

(b) Any direct measurement taken from a radiograph may be inaccurate as the image it depicts may be distorted by being shortened or lengthened. Also it does not take into account the length of the root of the tooth.

(c) $$\frac{\text{CEJ to bone crest (in mm)}}{\text{CEJ to root apex (in mm)}} \times 100$$

(d) Horizontal bone loss occurs when the base of the pocket lies coronal to the bony crest, creating a supra-bony pocket. Vertical bone loss is where more bone loss occurs on one side of the interdental bone crest than on the other. This leaves the base of the pocket within the bony defect and is an infra-bony pocket.

(e) Localised when < 30% of sites are affected or generalised when > 30% of sites are affected.

6.4 (a) What do you understand by the term cone-beam computed tomography (CBCT)?

(b) What are the main indications of CBCT?

(c) List two advantages and two disadvantages of CBCT.

Answer 6.4

(a) It is a three-dimensional digital radiographic image. A CT image is generated by a CT scanner using X-rays to produce a sectional or slice image of the body. The data are in a numerical (dicon) format and converted into a grey scale representing different tissue densities which generates an image. In conventional or medical CT the X-ray beam is fan shaped but in CBCT the beam is cone shaped.

(b) It can be used for any condition affecting the maxilla or mandible including:
- Cysts
- Tumours, both benign and malignant
- Antral disease (sinusitis/oroantral communication/foreign body/trauma/cyst/tumour/bony abnormalities or pathology)
- Bony abnormalities and pathology
- Implant assessment
- Temporomandibular joint imaging
- Assessment of unerupted/impacted teeth and odontomes
- Assessment of the relationship of the inferior alveolar/dental nerve to roots of a tooth, usually impacted third molars
- Orthodontic assessment
- Fractures of the facial bones
- Three-dimensional assessment of teeth and periodontal tissues.

(c) Advantages:
- Multiplanar imaging and manipulation so the anatomy can be seen in different planes
- Low radiation dose relative to conventional medical CT
- Fast scanning time
- Compatible with implant and cephalometric planning software
- Cheaper and smaller than conventional medical CT

Disadvantages:
- All information/data are obtained in a single scan so patient must remain stationary

- Soft tissue is not imaged in detail

- Artefacts from metal objects, eg restorations

- Reconstructed panoramic image is not directly comparable with the conventional dental panoramic radiograph

6.5 (a) What is tomography?

(b) How is this achieved?

(c) What is a focal trough?

(d) Give five indications for dental panoramic tomography.

(e) What do you understand by the term 'ghost shadows' with respect to dental panoramic tomography?

(f) What would an air shadow look like on a dental panoramic tomograph and why do they take on this appearance?

(g) What radiation dosage does a patient receive in this procedure?

Answer 6.5

(a) It is a technique for producing images of a slice or section of an object.

(b) The X-ray tube and the film cassette carrier are connected and move synchronously but in opposite directions about a pivoting point. The pivoting point will appear in focus on the radiograph.

(c) Only a slice of the object is in focus on the tomograph and this is called the focal trough.

(d) Any five of the following:
   • Assessment of third molars

   • Assessment for fractures of the mandible

   • To assess bone heights in periodontal disease with pockets greater than 5 mm in depth

   • Orthodontic assessment

   • To assess bony lesions of the mandible and maxilla

   • Implant planning

   • To assess bony disorders of the temporomandibular joints

   • To assess antral disease

(e) Ghost shadows are shadows cast by anatomical structures such as the cervical vertebrae and the mandible and palate, which are outside the focal trough on the panoramic radiograph. They appear on the opposite side of the real image counterpart and slightly higher up than the real image.

(f) Air shadows are radiolucent because there is no photon absorption whereas there is in tissue.

(g) 2.7–38 µSV depending on how the radiograph is taken.

6.6 (a) Name the error that could have occurred to produce the following faults in a panoramic radiograph.

   (i)   The film shows anterior teeth that are out of focus and magnified.

   (ii)   The molars are larger on one side than the other.

   (iii) There is vertical or horizontal distortion of one part of the image.

   (iv)   The radiograph is too dark.

   (b) What do you understand by the terms development and fixation with regard to radiographs?

Answer 6.6

(a) Errors producing the faults given in the question are:

   (i)   The patient is positioned too far from the film.

   (ii)   The patient has their head to one side or the other so they are asymmetrically positioned in the machine.

   (iii) The patient has moved while the radiograph was being taken.

   (iv)   There are several reasons:

   • Overexposure — due to increased exposure time either by operator error or faulty equipment

   • Overdevelopment — due to excessive time in the developer solution, the solution being too warm or too concentrated

   • Fogging — due to poor storage of the film or light leaking onto film during development

   • Patient with very thin tissues

(b) Development is when the sensitised silver halide crystals in the film emulsion are converted to metallic silver, which is black in colour and produces the black/grey part of the image. Fixation is when the unsensitised silver halide crystals on the film emulsion are removed. This produces the white/transparent part of the image.

6.7 (a) How often must a dentist attend a radiation protection update course?

(b) List five methods you could use to minimise the radiation dose to a patient having an intraoral radiograph.

(c) What do you understand by the term somatic stochastic effects of ionising radiation? What is the safe dose of ionising radiation to prevent these effects?

(d) How does ionising radiation damage the body?

(e) What is the estimated risk of developing fatal cancer from dental panoramic radiography?

Answer 6.7

(a) Five hours of radiation protection training every five years as part of continuing professional development

(b) Any five of the following:
- Justification

- High-speed film

- Rectangular collimation

- Quality control

- Optimal kilovoltage (70 kV)

- Digital radiography

- Aluminium filtration

- Rectification

- Use of film holders

- Appropriate focus to skin distance

(c) Stochastic means governed by the laws of probability or random. Hence stochastic effects are effects that may develop. There is no safe dose as they might occur after any dose of ionising radiation so every exposure carries the risk of stochastic effects. Obviously the lower the ionising radiation dose the lower the likelihood of damage, although the amount of damage is not related to the size of the inducing dose.

(d) The effects can cause direct or indirect damage. Direct damage involves ionising biological molecules, eg point mutations in DNA. Indirect damage occurs from ionising water, which leads to the formation of free radicals. These may combine to form highly reactive species which cause damage.

(e) 1:2 000 000

6.8 (a) From the right column of the table below select the most appropriate image to show the structures and conditions in the left column. Each option may be used once or not at all.

Structures/conditions	Image
A fractured zygomatic arch	Mandibular standard occlusal radiograph
Periodontal pocketing around lower incisors	Bitewing radiographs
Interproximal caries	10° occipitomental radiograph
Internal derangement of the temporomandibular joint	CT scan of the face
An impacted lower third molar	Long cone periapical radiographs
A fluid level in the maxillary antrum	Bisecting angle periapical radiographs
A blow-out fracture of the orbital floor	MR scan
A salivary calculus in the submandibular duct	Submentovertex radiograph
Presence of an impacted permanent upper canine	Maxillary standard occlusal radiograph
	Panoramic radiograph
	Reverse Townes' radiograph

Answer 6.8

Structures/conditions	Image
A fractured zygomatic arch	Submentovertex radiograph
Periodontal pocketing around lower incisors	Long cone periapical radiographs
Interproximal caries	Bitewing radiographs
Internal derangement of the temporomandibular joint	MR scan
An impacted lower third molar	Panoramic radiograph
A fluid level in the maxillary antrum	10° occipitomental radiograph
A blow-out fracture of the orbital floor	CT scan of the face
A salivary calculus in the submandibular duct	Mandibular standard occlusal radiograph
Presence of an impacted permanent upper canine	Maxillary standard occlusal radiograph

Submental vertex radiograph gives the best view of fractured zygomatic arch but is now rarely done; to reduce the radiation dose to patient two occipitomental radiographs are usually taken.

6.9 (a) What do you understand by the ALARP principle?

(b) List seven factors that can help achieve this principle.

(c) Should lead aprons be used routinely in dental radiography? Please give a reason for your answer.

(d) What are the annual dose limits of radiation for non-classified workers?

Answer 6.9

(a) ALARP is an acronym that stands for 'as low as reasonably practicable' and is meant to minimise exposure to radiation.

(b) Any seven of the following:
- Every radiograph must be justified.

- All exposures should be kept as low as reasonably practicable — they should be optimised.

- There should be limitation of radiation dose.

- There should be written guidelines for exposure setting for radiographs.

- The fastest speed film should be used that will give a good quality image (usually E).

- A rectangular collimator should be used.

- There should be minimal skin to focus distances (> 60 kV = 20 cm).

- Film holders should be used rather than patients holding the film.

- When referring a patient the radiographs should be sent with the patient to avoid further radiation.

- All radiographs should be evaluated and an entry made in the patient's notes.

- There should be a quality assurance programme in place to optimise results.

(c) There is no justification for the routine use of lead aprons in dental radiography as reducing radiation is best achieved by implementing measures such as clinical judgement, equipment optimisation and radiographic technique. This is given in the *Guidance Notes for Dental Practitioners on the Safe Use of X-ray Equipment* published in 2001 by the Department of Health.

(d) 6 mSv

6.10 (a) What is sialography? Give two indications and contraindications for using it.

(b) Submandibular duct salivary calculi/obstructions can sometimes be seen on routine radiography. On which radiographic views would you see submandibular duct salivary calculi?

(c) Ultrasound can be used for imaging salivary glands. Give four advantages of using ultrasound for this purpose.

Answer 6.10

(a) Sialography involves introducing a radiopaque medium into the ductal system of a major salivary gland and then taking a radiographic image.

Indications:
- Obstructions in the ductal system, eg calculi

- It is used to assess the structure of the gland and ductal system and to see if there is any destruction or changes in them.

Contraindications — any two of the following:
- Allergy to iodine-containing compounds

- Infection in the gland

- A calculus close to the duct orifice which may be pushed further back by the introduction of contrast medium.

(b) Dental panoramic radiograph and lower standard occlusal

(c) Any four of the following:
- No ionising radiation used

- Excellent for superficial masses

- Can use it to guide fine needle aspiration

- Can use to differentiate between solid and cystic masses

- It can identify radiolucent calculi not seen on radiographs.

- It can be used to break up calculi by lithotripsy.

- Intraoral masses can be visualised with small probes.

6.11 (a) Describe what a keratocystic odontogenic tumour (odontogenic keratocyst) may look like on a radiograph.

(b) Describe what a dentigerous cyst may look like on a radiograph.

(c) If a patient had a lesion at the angle of their mandible what radiographic views could be taken to demonstrate it and what would each view show?

Answer 6.11

(a) Radiographic features of a keratocystic odontogenic tumour:
  • Radiolucent lesion

  • Well defined

  • Multilocular although may be unilocular

  • Rounded margins

  • Adjacent teeth may be displaced

  • Tooth roots are not usually resorbed

(b) Radiographic features of a dentigerous cyst:
  • Radiolucent lesion

  • Well circumscribed

  • Usually unilocular but there may be pseudo-loculation due to bony trabeculae

  • Rounded

  • Contains the crown of a tooth, or lies adjacent to the crown of a tooth

  • Associated tooth is usually displaced

(c) A dental panoramic radiograph, sectional dental panoramic tomograph or oblique lateral views would show the lesion. The mesiodistal and superior/inferior dimensions of the lesion would be evident as well as association with any teeth, the inferior dental canal, etc. A posterior–anterior (PA) view of the mandible will show any buccolingual expansion of the mandible.

6.12 (a) One technique for taking periapical radiographs is the paralleling technique. Name another technique.

(b) Give an advantage of using this technique compared with the paralleling technique.

(c) What are the advantages of using a paralleling technique in periapical radiography?

(d) Describe how you would set up the tube head to take a bitewing radiograph and why.

Answer 6.12

(a) Bisecting angle technique

(b) Any one of the following:
- Positioning of the film packet in any area of the mouth is usually more comfortable for the patient.

- It is straightforward and quick.

- The length of the crowns and roots should be the same as the teeth being radiographed if the film and tube have been correctly positioned.

(c) Advantages of using a paralleling technique:
- There is no image distortion.

- Images are reproducible at different visits and with different operators.

- There is no 'coning off' of the image.

- Rectangular collimation will reduce the radiation dose to patients.

- Periodontal bone levels and the crowns of teeth are well shown.

- There is no superimposition of the zygomatic buttress on the maxillary molars.

(d) The X-ray beam is angled downwards by 5–8° to account for the curve of Monson on the occlusal plane. It is also aimed through the contact points at right angles to the teeth and the film packet to avoid overlap of the contact areas.

6.13 (a) When taking a radiograph a certain part of the room is designated as controlled area. What do you understand by this term?

(b) How large is this area? Give an example of the radius for a machine taking panoramic dental radiographs and intraoral periapicals.

(c) What measures are advised with regard to the above?

(d) Digital radiography is becoming more popular. What is used instead of a film packet when taking a digital radiograph?

(e) Give four advantages of digital radiography over conventional radiography.

Answer 6.13

(a) The controlled area is within the primary beam until it has gone far enough to be reduced in strength or gone through shielding. It also includes the area around the patient and X-ray tube.

(b) The size of the area depends on the voltage of the equipment. For an intraoral radiograph the radius is 1 m and for a panoramic radiograph it is 1.5 (as panoramic machines have a peak operating potential greater than 70 kVp).

(c) Hazard lights which should be illuminated during the exposure, and signs on the door are needed.

(d) A charged couple device (CCD), a complementary metal oxide semiconductor, a photostimulable phosphor imaging plate (PSPP)

(e) Any four of the following:
- No processing faults

- No risk from handling the chemicals involved in processing

- Lower radiation dose as the image receptors are more sensitive than conventional film

- Ease of storage of images

- Ease of transfer of images

- Electronic enhancement of images

6.14

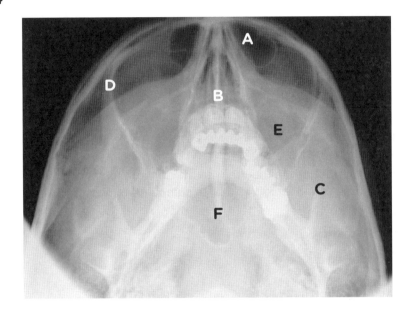

(a) What view is shown in the figure?

(b) Give four indications for taking this view.

(c) What can you see on this view?

(d) Indicate the structures labelled A—F?

Answer 6.14

(a) Occipito-mental view (30°)

(b) Any four of the following:
- Suspected fracture of the zygomatic complex
- Middle third facial injuries
- Le Fort I, II, III fractures
- Nasoethmoidal complex fractures
- Orbital fractures (although with the above, except for zygomatic fractures, other imaging such as computed tomography is also often done).
- Coronoid process fractures
- Frontal sinus and ethmoidal sinus visualisation

(c) Fracture of the right zygomatic complex with disruption at the inferior orbital rim and the zygomatic buttress

(d)

A: frontal sinus

B: nasal septum

C: coronoid process

D: lateral orbital margin

E: maxillary antrum

F: sphenoidal sinus

6.15   A 30-year-old man was injured in a road traffic accident. He was taken by ambulance to accident and emergency. On examination he had sustained head injury and a laceration. He is conscious with no focal neurological signs.

fig. 1

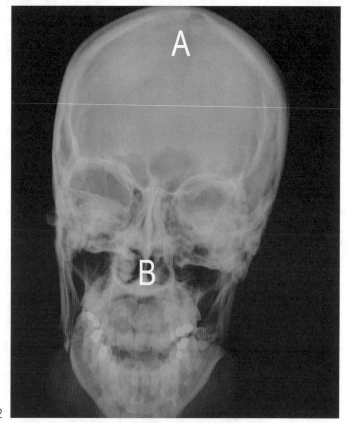

fig. 2

(a) What view is shown in fig. 1?

(b) What abnormality is seen on this radiograph?

(c) If you wanted more information about the orbital fracture which type of image would you order?

(d) A similar image can be used if a patient had an orbital floor fracture. What is often seen on the image?

(e) A similar radiograph is shown in fig. 2. What abnormality is seen in the mandible?

(f) Which radiographic view would give you a better view of this abnormality?

(g) What are the structures labelled A and B in fig. 2?

Answer 6.15

(a) PA view of the skull

(b) Fracture of his frontal bone/superior orbital margin

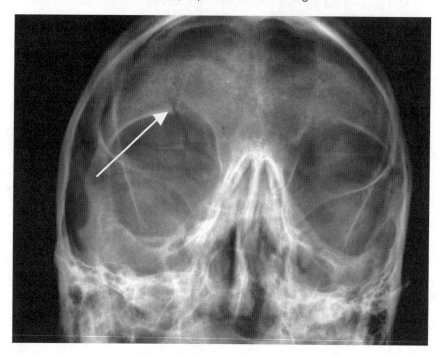

(c) A CT scan

(d) Herniation of orbital contents into the maxillary antrum.

(e) Fracture of the right angle of the mandible

(f) It would be identified better on a PA view of the jaws/mandible, a panoramic radiograph or an oblique lateral view.

(g)

- A: sagittal suture

- B: inferior turbinate

6.16 (a) Describe what you can see on the radiograph shown in the figure.

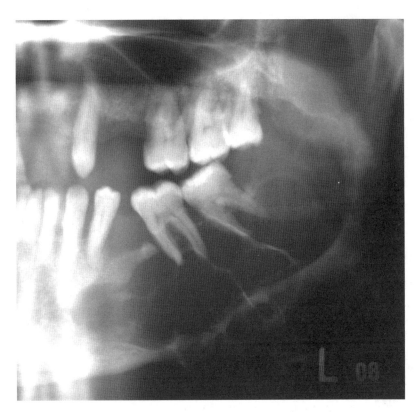

(b) What is your differential diagnosis?

(c) The inferior dental canal is seen on this view. How might the inferior dental canal look on a radiograph if it was associated with an impacted wisdom tooth?

Answer 6.16

(a) A radiolucent area at the angle and body of left side of the mandible. It extends from the first premolar to the ascending ramus of the mandible. It is multilocular with distinct septa. The outline is smooth, scalloped and well defined, and there are internal septa. There is bony expansion of the mandible and displacement of inferior dental canal. There is no resorption of the tooth roots.

(b) Differential diagnosis:
- Ameloblastoma
- Keratocystic odontogenic tumour (odontogenic keratocyst)
- Calcifying epithelial odontogenic tumour (early stage)
- Myxoma
- Ameloblastic fibroma
- Haemangioma

(c)
- Narrowing of the tramlines
- Deviation of the tramlines
- Loss of the tramlines
- Radiolucent banding across the root

7
Human Disease and Therapeutics

7.1 The following patients all take different drugs that interfere with some aspect of clotting. How would your management differ for each of the cases if you needed to extract a tooth for them?

1 Patient 1 takes warfarin for atrial fibrillation.

2 Patient 2 takes aspirin after a myocardial infarction.

3 Patient 3 takes aspirin and clopidrogrel after placement of a cardiac stent.

4 Patient 4 takes aspirin and dipyridamole for stroke prevention.

5 Patient 5 takes dabigatran etexilate (a thrombin inhibitor) for atrial fibrillation.

Answer 7.1

1 Patients on warfarin need to have an international normalised ratio (INR) check done within 72 h of the extraction; if they have an unstable INR this time interval drops to 24 h. If the INR falls within the range 1—4, it is deemed safe to carry out the extraction. (Care should be taken at the upper end of this range, especially if multiple teeth or surgical procedures may be necessary.) Local measures should also be employed such as packing the socket with a haemostatic agent, eg oxidised cellulose or collagen sponge, or resorbable gelatin sponge, and the socket should be sutured. Good postoperative instructions should be given and non-steroidal anti-inflammatory drugs (NSAIDs) should not be prescribed. Postoperative tranexamic acid mouthwash may also be considered

2 Patient 2 takes aspirin and usually extractions can be carried out without any ill effect. If excessive bleeding occurs on removal of the tooth, it would be prudent to pack and suture the socket as in patient 1 and prescription of NSAIDs should be avoided

3 Clopidrogrel and aspirin may cause postoperative bleeding, so it is good practice to pack and suture all sockets as in patient 1. The prescription of NSAIDs should be avoided, but postoperative tranexamic acid mouthwash may be considered. There is no preoperative blood test that is recommended

4 Dipyridamole and aspirin are a less potent combination than clopidrogrel and aspirin, and patients can be safely managed in the same manner as those on aspirin alone

5 Dabigatran etexilate is a new thrombin inhibitor. It differs from warfarin in that vitamin K is not an effective reversal agent, and the drug's action is not monitored by measuring the INR. It has a much shorter half-life of 12—17 h, but this depends on renal activity. In patients with poor renal function the half-life is increased

As there are no guidelines at present on how to manage patients on these drugs who require surgical procedures in dentistry, it would be sensible to liaise with the patient's haematologist about management. It would seem prudent to check the patient's renal function if possible because this will give an indication of the drug's half-life. It is also suggested that the patient should be treated as late as is feasibly possibly after administration of the drug, eg if the patient takes it at night, then treat the following afternoon. Local measures such as packing, suturing and postoperative administration of tranexamic acid mouthwash are also suggested

7.2 (a) What features would lead you to suspect alcohol dependency in a patient?

(b) What is the current recommendation for alcohol intake in the UK?

(c) What are the complications of excessive alcohol intake and how may excessive alcohol intake affect your management of a dental patient?

Answer 7.2

(a) Alcohol abuse and dependence are now both included under the diagnosis alcohol use disorder. It is a disease that is characterised by the person having a pattern of excessive drinking despite the negative effects of alcohol on the individual's work, medical, legal, educational and/or social life. It may involve a destructive pattern of alcohol use including a number of symptoms, such as tolerance to or withdrawal from the substance, use of more alcohol and/or for a longer time than planned, and trouble reducing its use. Alcohol abuse is on the less severe end of the alcohol use disorder spectrum whereas alcohol dependency is on the more severe end of the spectrum.

The following are characteristic of alcohol dependency:
   * Tolerance — the need to drink more and more alcohol to feel the same effects

   * Withdrawal symptoms — this occurs after stopping or cutting back on drinking; symptoms are anxiety, sweating, trembling, trouble sleeping, nausea or vomiting, and, in severe cases, physical seizures and hallucinations

   * Preoccupation with drinking

   * Paying less attention to other life activities (primacy)

   * Persisting with substance use despite clear evidence of being overtly harmful

   * A strong desire or sense of compulsion to take the substance; loss of control

The patient may come in smelling of alcohol or appear to be under the influence of alcohol.

(b) There is no safe limit for alcohol intake.
   * The UK guidelines for alcohol state that men should not regularly drink more than 3—4 units per day and women more than 2—3 units per day.

   * 'Regularly' means drinking most days or every day.

   * Men should drink no more than 21 units per week.

   * Women should drink no more than 14 units per week.

- There should be at least two alcohol-free days per week.

1 unit = 10 ml/8 g or pure alcohol = 25 ml spirit = 175-ml glass of wine.

In the USA, the Centers for Disease Control and Prevention state: heavy drinking for men is typically defined as consuming 15 drinks or more per week, and for women as consuming 8 drinks or more per week.

(c) Excessive and prolonged alcohol consumption can lead to:
- Liver disease and cirrhosis which can cause a bleeding tendency and problems with drug metabolism

- Gastrointestinal tract: gastritis and oesophagitis, so limits use of NSAIDs

- Cardiovascular system: hypertension, cardiomyopathy, risk of arrhythmia and potential concern with use of local anaesthetic

- Central nervous system: poor comprehension, potential issues with consent

- Poor compliance

Avoid metronidazole use because it may cause a disulfiram-type reaction.

7.3 (a) How would you define obesity?

(b) What physical difficulties may you encounter when carrying out dental treatment in an obese patient?

(c) What are the other dental relevances of obesity?

Answer 7.3

(a) The World Health Organization (WHO) defines obesity as 'Abnormal or excessive fat accumulation that may impair health'. The current definition of obesity by the WHO and the US National Institutes of Health is a BMI (body mass index) ≥ 30 kg/m^2.

- Waist circumference: in addition to measuring BMI, circumference measurements are also used in overweight and obese adults to assess abdominal obesity. A waist circumference ≥ 40 inches (102 cm) for men and ≥ 35 inches (88 cm) for women is considered elevated and indicative of increased cardiometabolic risk (Jensen et al, 2014 *Circulation*). Waist circumference measurement is unnecessary in patients with BMI ≥ 35 kg/m^2, because almost all individuals with this BMI will also have an abnormal waist circumference and are at a high risk from their obesity.

Obesity, a chronic disease that is increasing in prevalence in adults, adolescents and children, is now considered to be a global epidemic. Obesity is associated with a significant increase in mortality and risk of many disorders, including diabetes mellitus, hypertension, dyslipidaemia, heart disease, stroke, sleep apnoea, cancer and others.

Note: the definitions of overweight and obesity vary by race.

(b)

- Access for dental treatment may be affected.
- The patient may not be able to travel to the practice or get into the building or room due to the size of the doors or stairwell.
- Special bariatric chairs may be necessary (maximum lifting weight for modern chairs is approximately 140 kg/23 stone).
- The patient may not be able to lie down supine.
- Blood pressure cuffs may be too small and hence give an incorrect reading.

(c)

- Landmarks for giving inferior dental blocks may be difficult to determine due to the volume of tissue.

- Managing a medical emergency may be difficult — intravenous cannulation may be more difficult to achieve.

- Intramuscular injection may be less predicable due to injection into fat rather than muscle as a result of tissue bulk.

- Airway management is also potentially more difficult.

These factors should be considered in the conscious sedation of obese patients, so consider referral of such cases to secondary care.

Obese individuals may have a higher incidence of infection and delayed wound healing. Obesity impairs the cell-mediated immune responses and decreases lymphocyte immune function and natural killer T-cell activity.

- Diabetes: >80% of cases of type 2 diabetes mellitus can be attributed to obesity (timing for dental treatment, hypoglycaemia, risk of infection).

- Hypertension: persistent obesity not only raises the blood pressure directly, but also makes the hypertension more difficult to control by interfering with the efficacy of antihypertensive drugs (ischaemic heart disease, lichenoid reaction due to antihypertensive agents).

- Heart disease: obesity is associated with a number of risk factors for cardiovascular disease, including hypertension, insulin resistance and diabetes mellitus, and dyslipidaemia. Obesity is also associated with increased risks of coronary disease and heart failure.

- Heart failure: there is an important association between obesity and heart failure — patient unable to lie flat for treatment.

- Atrial fibrillation/flutter: obese individuals are significantly more likely to develop atrial fibrillation (anticoagulant).

- Stroke: obesity is associated with an increased risk of stroke.

- Respiratory system: there is increased risk of obstructive sleep apnoea in obesity, so may need to be managed with mandibular advancement device, continuous positive airway pressure (CPAP) with associated dry mouth or even orthognathic surgery.

- General anaesthesia implications: increasing obesity leads to respiratory and cardiovascular changes that have an impact on the delivery of anaesthesia and perioperative analgesia. Bariatric beds and patient transfer devices are unsuitable for day surgery.

Pharmacology: Modified drug dosing is required for GA and other drugs. *British Dental Journal* 2009; **207**:171–5.

7.4 (a) When assessing an unwell patient we follow the ABCDE approach. What does each of these letters stand for?

(b) Briefly describe how you would assess the A and B components in an unwell adult patient in your dental practice.

Answer 7.4

(a) Airway, Breathing, Circulation, Disability, Exposure.

(b)

A — Airway
- *Speak* to the patient and ask them if they are all right. If they can respond and talk to you then their airway is patent.

- Airway obstruction may be partial or complete. Partial obstruction tends to cause noisy breathing, whereas in complete obstruction there are no breath sounds, hence *listening to the breath sounds* will give a clue as to where the problem is.

- If the obstruction is in the lower airways, there is usually a wheeze on expiration.

- If the obstruction is in the larynx or above, there is usually stridor on inspiration.

- Material such as liquid or semi-solids in the upper airway will cause gurgling.

- If the pharynx is partially blocked by the tongue or palate then there will be snoring.

- *Observe* the patient trying to breathe as in airway obstruction as the patient struggles to breathe they will use their accessory muscles of respiration in the neck and there may well be a see-saw movement of the chest and abdomen. Cyanosis of the lips and tongue will occur as a late sign.

B — Breathing
- Following the ABCDE approach you would only assess this once you had completed assessing A, so you would have all the information from A already.

- Count the respiratory rate, the normal is 12–20 breaths per minute and below 5 or above 36 is serious.

- Assess whether both sides of the chest are moving equally and the depth and pattern of breathing.

- If you have a pulse oximeter available in your practice you could use this to assess the oxygen saturation levels.

- It is not common for dental practitioners to be highly skilled at listening to breath sounds with a stethoscope or have a stethoscope available in the dental practice. However, if the equipment is available and the individual is skilled, the chest should be auscultated.

For further information on the ABDCE approach, see www.resus.org.uk.

7.5 (a) What do you understand by the term immunocompromised?

(b) In the list below, which are primary (innate) conditions and which are secondary (acquired) conditions that cause a patient to be immunocompromised:

- Autoimmune: systemic lupus erythematosus (SLE)
- Chédiak–Higashi syndrome
- Drug induced
- Human immunodeficiency virus (HIV) infection
- Leukocyte adhesion defect type I/(LAD1)
- Malignancies: leukaemias, Hodgkin's disease
- Papillon–Lefèvre syndrome
- Selective IgA disease

(c) Why might a patient be given immunosuppressive drugs?

(d) What are the oral signs that might present in an immunocompromised patient?

(e) What tests would you want to carry out to determine a patient's immune function prior to extraction of a lower molar?

Answer 7.5

(a) Immunocompromised — the immune function of a patient is inherently poor. It can be suppressed artificially or depressed due to illness and they may be at risk of concurrent illness due to the reduced function of the immune system.

(b)

Primary conditions:
- Selective IgA disease
- Chédiak–Higashi syndrome
- Papillon Lefèvre syndrome
- LAD1

Secondary conditions:
- HIV
- Malignancies: leukaemias, Hodgkin's disease
- Autoimmune: SLE
- Drug induced

(c)

- Anti-rejection therapy for organ transplantation
- To treat autoimmune conditions
- To treat connective tissue disorders
- Control some lymphoproliferative tumours

(d)

- Oral ulceration
- Mucositis
- Oral infections — bacterial, viral and fungal
- Xerostomia
- Hairy tongue

(e) You would check the levels of their white blood cells (WBCs) to ensure that they were able to resist infection. Hence you would want to check the WBC count:

Normal: 4.5–10 × 10^9 /l

Differential white cell count:
- Lymphocytes 1–3.5 × 10^9 /l
- CD4 and CD8
    - CD4 500–1500/mm^3
    - CD8 230–750/mm^3
    - Ratio CD4:CD8 = 1.2–3.8
- Neutrophils 2.0–7.5 × 10^9 /l
- Monocytes 0.2–0.8 × 10^9 /l
- Eosinophils 0.04–0.44 × 10^9 /l
- Basophils 0–0.1 × 10^9 /1

7.6   (a) What is the cause of Down syndrome?

(b) Name three orodental features that a patient with Down syndrome may have.

(c) What are the implications of Down syndrome on the delivery of oral healthcare?

(d) How would you gain consent from a patient with Down syndrome to carry out invasive dental treatment if the patient was aged 19?

Answer 7.6

(a) A genetic condition caused by trisomy of chromosome 21.

(b)

- Hypodontia/microdontia
- Delayed development and delayed eruption of both deciduous and permanent teeth
- Hypocalcification/hypoplastic defects
- Early onset periodontal disease
- Gingivitis on anterior teeth due to mouth breathing
- Anterior open bite, posterior crossbite and class III incisor relationship

(c)

- Learning disability, although the degree varies from person to person
- Cardiac abnormalities, some requiring surgical correction
- Visual problems such as cataracts
- Auditory problems due to fluid accumulation in the middle ear
- Joints — atlanto-axial joint instability — do not hyper-extend the neck
- Compromised immune system — increased susceptibility to infections (bacterial/viral/fungal)
- Neurological conditions — epilepsy — management, drugs — gingival hyperplasia, sugar containing drugs, dry mouth
- Alzheimer's disease

(d) You would consent the patient in the same way that you would consent any 19 year old. You would assess the patient's understanding of the issues prudent to gaining consent. If they were competent and understood everything then you can proceed as normal. If they do not understand or are not competent then no one else can consent for the patient. However, it is usually good practice to get agreement from the patient's carers or family, but they cannot consent for them. Treatment must be deemed to be in the best interest of the patient, and in that situation two healthcare professionals (doctor/dentist) must agree on the treatment. However, if emergency treatment is needed then this can be carried out rather than delay the treatment while waiting to find a second healthcare professional.

7.7 (a) What is the mechanism of action of the following autoimmune
             reactions? Give an example of each.

   - Type I

   - Type II

   - Type III

   - Type IV

  (b) What signs and symptoms might a patient experiencing a type I
       reaction show?

  (c) Latex allergy is common in the general population. Name six items
       in a dental surgery that may contain latex.

Answer 7.7

(a) Mechanism of action and any one of the examples given:
- Type I — immediate reaginic (anaphylaxis, allergic asthma, allergic rhinitis)

- Type II — antibody dependent (transfusion reactions, myasthenia gravis)

- Type III — immune complex (rheumatoid arthritis, systemic lupus erythematosus)

- Type IV — cell mediated (contact dermatitis, pemphigoid, Hashimoto's thyroiditis)

(b) Rash, itching, facial flushing, tingling of face, swelling of tongue, wheeze, stridor, collapse

(c) Any six of the following:
- Local anaesthetic cartridges

- Examination and surgical gloves

- Rubber dam

- Mouth props

- Anaesthetic masks and hoses

- Blood pressure cuffs

- Orthodontic elastics

- Mixing bowls

- Endodontic stops

Latex-free alternatives are available.

7.8 (a) What type of drug is warfarin and what is its mode of action?

(b) How is warfarin treatment monitored?

(c) List three medical conditions for which patients may be prescribed warfarin.

(d) Which of the following drugs may interact with warfarin? Do they enhance or decrease the action of the warfarin?

- Fluconazole
- Penicillin
- Metronidazole
- Adrenaline/epinephrine
- Paracetamol
- Carbemazepine

(e) What type of drug is tranexamic acid? How is it administered and when would it be used?

Answer 7.8

(a) Warfarin is an anticoagulant, and it is a vitamin K antagonist.

(b) By measuring a patient's INR (international normalised ratio), which is the ratio of patient's prothrombin time to control prothrombin time

(c) Any three of the following:
- Atrial fibrillation
- Prosthetic heart valves
- Deep vein thrombosis
- Pulmonary embolus
- Cerebrovascular accident
- Antiphospholipid syndrome

(d) Drugs that interact with warfarin:
- Fluconazole — enhances anticoagulant effect
- Metronidazole — enhances anticoagulant effect
- Carbamazepine — reduces anticoagulant effect

(e) Tranexamic acid is an antifibrinolytic agent. It may be used topically as a mouthwash or by soaking swabs in it and getting the patient to bite on them. It can also be given orally or intravenously. It is used to prevent and control bleeding especially during and after the procedure.

7.9 What are the dental implications of the following findings in a patient's medical history:

(a) The patient is taking glyceryl trinitrate (GTN).

(b) The patient is taking Insulatard.

(c) The patient is taking nifedipine.

(d) The patient has had infective endocarditis in the past but is not allergic to penicillin.

(e) The patient has osteoporosis and is taking biphosphonate tablets (Fosamax™ 70mg) once a week.

Answer 7.9

(a) GTN is a vasodilator and also reduces left ventricular work by reducing venous return. Hence it is used to provide symptomatic relief in angina. Angina occurs when there is an imbalance between the demand and supply of blood to the heart and the patient experiences crushing central chest pain that can radiate down the left arm. An attack may be precipitated by dental treatment. Reducing stress by providing good anaesthesia and not subjecting patients to long appointments will minimise the likelihood of the patient having an attack. In addition, the patient should take GTN at the start of an appointment.

(b) Insulatard is an insulin preparation that is used to control the blood glucose levels in patients with type 1 diabetes mellitus. Patients self-administer Insulatard subcutaneously. Diabetic patients have poor wound healing and are more susceptible to infections. Hence they are prone to gingivitis, rapidly progressing periodontal disease and oral candidal infections. They may also have xerostomia. Treatment should be timed so that it does not interfere with the meal times as hypoglycaemia may develop and the patient may collapse.

(c) Nifedipine is a calcium-channel blocker used to treat hypertension. Hypertensive patients are at increased risk of other cardiovascular disease. Routine dental treatment may need to be postponed if the patient's blood pressure is greater than 160/110 mmHg. Hypertensive patients are more likely to have excessive bleeding following extractions. Nifedipine can cause gingival hyperplasia.

(d) Patients who have had previous infective endocarditis are no longer given antibiotic cover prior to dental treatment (see Answer 7.23). It is thought that maintaining a good standard of oral hygiene and dental health is more important as a bacteraemia can occur following chewing and tooth brushing, and not just invasive dental treatment.

(e) Patients who take bisphosphonates are at greater risk of getting medication-related osteonecrosis of the jaws (MRONJ). This may arise spontaneously or following dental treatment, especially extractions. In terms of dental treatment it is important to make sure that dentures fit well and are relined if necessary as trauma may lead to MRONJ. Routine dental treatment can be carried out with little likelihood of risk. Extractions may cause MRONJ, however, the risk is very low, and hence it may be advisable to restore teeth rather than extract if possible. If extractions cannot be avoided then patients should be informed about the risk when consent is to be gained and it may be advisable to give the patient pre- and postoperative chlorhexidine mouthwash. It may also be advisable to limit extractions to one quadrant at a time and wait for sockets to heal fully before moving on to the next quadrant.

7.10 Which drug, dose and route (see first table, below) should be used in the emergencies listed in the second table, below? Choose the most appropriate from the options given below. Each option may be used once, more than once or not at all.

Drugs	Dosage	Route
Adrenaline/epinephrine	10 mg	Buccal
Diclofenac	1 g	Intravenous
Glucose	100 mg	Intramuscular
Glyceryl trinitrate	0.5 ml of 1:1000	Oral
Insulin	5 ml of a 50% solution	PR
Nitrous oxide/oxygen	50 ml of a 50% solution	Subcutaneous
Salbutamol	2 puffs/nebuliser	Sublingual

Emergency	Drugs	Dosage	Route
Anaphylaxis			
Hypoglycaemic collapse			
Status epilepticus			
Myocardial infarction			
Asthmatic attack			

Answer 7.10

Emergency	Drug	Dose	Route
Anaphylaxis	Adrenaline/ epinephrine	0.5–1 ml of 1:1000	Intramuscular
Hypoglycaemic collapse	Glucose	50 ml of a 50% solution	Intravenous
Status epilepticus	Midazdam	10 mg	Buccal
Myocardial infarction	Nitrous oxide/ oxygen		Inhalational
Asthmatic attack	Salbutamol	2 puffs/nebuliser	Inhalational

7.11 (a) What do the following terms mean?

- Autograft

- Allograft

- Xenograft

(b) Give an example of each.

(c) Many patients who receive transplants are on immunosuppressant medication. What are the side effects of immunosuppressant medication?

(d) Ciclosporin is a commonly used immunosuppressant drug. Name a complication that can occur with its use.

(e) Name another commonly used immunosuppressant drug.

Answer 7.11

(a)
- Autograft — from the same person
- Allograft — from an individual of the same species
- Xenograft — from a different species

(b) Examples:
- Autograft — iliac crest bone to jaw
- Allograft — kidney, liver, cornea, heart, lung
- Xenograft — porcine heart valves

(c) Side effects of immunosuppressants:
- Increased risk of infection
- Increased risk of cancer (skin and haematological)

(d) Any one of the following:
- Gingival hyperplasia
- Diabetes
- Hypertension

(e) Any one of the following:
- Azathioprine
- Mycophenolate

7.12 (a) What are the major systemic side effects of steroids? List four of the systems that may be affected and give two examples of each.

(b) Name an oral condition for which a patient may be prescribed topical steroids.

(c) Name a head and neck condition for which a patient may be prescribed systemic steroids.

Answer 7.12

(a) Any four of the following systems and any two of the following examples:
- Gastrointestinal — peptic ulceration, dyspepsia, oesophageal candidal infection

- Musculoskeletal — proximal myopathy, osteoporosis, vertebral and long bone fractures

- Endocrine — adrenal suppression, Cushing syndrome, hirsutism, weight gain, increased appetite and increased susceptibility to infection

- Neuro-psychiatric — mood changes, depression, euphoria, psychological dependence psychosis

- Eye — glaucoma, increased intraocular pressure

- Skin — skin atrophy, telangiectasia, bruising and acne

(b) Any one of the following:
- Recurrent aphthous ulceration

- Lichen planus

(c) Any one of the following:
- Bell's palsy

- Giant cell arteritis

- Pemphigoid

- Pemphigus

- Sarcoidosis

7.13 (a) What causes HIV disease?

(b) How does it spread?

(c) What part of the immune response is affected?

(d) Name five oral conditions/lesions strongly associated with HIV disease.

(e) What types of drug are used to treat HIV disease?

(f) What is the importance of HIV for a dentist?

Answer 7.13

(a) HIV disease is caused by infection with human immunodeficiency viruses, which are RNA retroviruses.

(b) HIV infection can be transmitted:
- Sexually
- Through blood and blood products
- Intravenous drug misuse
- From mother to child

(c) T-cell-mediated immunity, in particular, CD4-positive lymphocytes.

(d) Any five of the following:
- Kaposi's sarcoma
- Candidal infections
- Hairy leukoplakia
- Periodontal disease (gingivitis and periodontitis)
- Non-Hodgkin's lymphoma
- Necrotising ulcerative gingivitis
- Ulcers

(e) Drugs used to treat HIV disease:
- Nucleoside reverse transcriptase inhibitors and non-nucleoside reverse transcriptase inhibitors
- Protease inhibitors

(f) There is risk of cross-infection. The patient is immunocompromised and hence may be more susceptible to infection than a healthy patient. They would be on multidrug treatment.

7.14 (a) How is liver disease relevant to dentistry?

(b) How are the following diseases spread?
- Hepatitis A
- Hepatitis B
- Hepatitis C
- Hepatitis D

(c) What infective agent causes hepatitis B?

(d) Which type of hepatitis can people be vaccinated against?

(e) Which type of hepatitis must all dental personnel be vaccinated against?

(f) What type of vaccine is used in (e)?

Answer 7.14

(a) Relevance of liver disease to dentistry:
- Patients with liver disease may have excess bleeding because of abnormal clotting factors.
- Patients with liver disease may be unable to metabolise drugs normally.
- Patients with liver disease may have a transmissible disease that could be a potential cross-infection risk.
- Patients may have delayed healing due to hypoproteinaemia and hence immunoglobulin deficiency.
- Administration of intravenous sedation may result in coma.

(b) Mode of spread of hepatitis:
- Hepatitis A — orofaecal
- Hepatitis B — parental, sexually and perinatally
- Hepatitis C — parental, sexually and perinatally
- Hepatitis D — parental, sexually and perinatally

(c) A DNA virus called hepatitis B virus

(d) A and B

(e) Hepatitis B

(f) Recombinant DNA hepatitis surface antigen (HbsAg)

7.15 (a) Match the drug with the appropriate statement.

Aciclovir	Inactivated by gastric acid and is best given by injections
Amphotericin	Active against many streptococci
Benzylpenicillin	Active against β-lactamase producing bacteria as it contains clavulanic acid
Co-amoxiclav	May cause pseudomembranous colitis
Clindamycin	Associated with 'red man' syndrome
Metronidazole	Active against anaerobes
Phenoxymethylpenicillin	Is a polyene antifungal drug
Vancomycin	Can be used to treat herpes simplex infections

(b) Give four indications of systemic antibiotics in dentistry.

Answer 7.15

(a)

Aciclovir	Can be used to treat herpes simplex infections
Amphotericin	Is a polyene antifungal drug
Benzylpenicillin	Inactivated by gastric acid and is best given by injections
Co-amoxiclav	Active against β-lactamase producing bacteria due to containing clavulanic acid
Clindamycin	May cause pseudomembranous colitis
Metronidazole	Active against anaerobes
Phenoxymethylpenicillin	Active against many streptococci
Vancomycin	Associated with 'red man' syndrome

(b) Indications for systemic antibiotics in dentistry:

- Treatment of spreading infection

- Prevention of postoperative infection

- Antibiotic cover to prevent infection in patients who have taken intravenous biphosphonate, anti-resorptive or anti-angiogenesis drugs or those that have had radiotherapy to the jaws (although this is not universally accepted, and local guidelines may vary)

- Prevention of infection following oral and maxillofacial trauma

7.16 (a) What do you understand by the term anaemia?

(b) What clinical features other than oral symptoms may the patient have?

(c) What oral conditions may anaemia predispose to?

(d) What is sickle cell disease?

(e) Which group of patients is most likely to be affected?

(f) When is it of concern to a dentist?

Answer 7.16

(a) Anaemia is a reduction in the oxygen-carrying capacity of the blood. It is defined by a low value for haemoglobin (females < 115 g/l and males <135 g/l).

(b) Symptoms vary with severity of the anaemia and range from pallor, fatigue, weakness, breathlessness, tachycardia and palpitations, dizziness, tinnitus, vertigo, headache and dyspnoea (shortness of breath) on exertion to angina, cardiac failure and gastrointestinal disturbances.

(c) Anaemia predisposes to:
- Glossitis

- Candidal infections and angular cheilitis

- Recurrent aphthae

(d) Sickle cell disease is an autosomal recessive condition in which there is a defect in a haemoglobin chain, which can cause haemolysis and anaemia. At low oxygen tensions or acidaemia the abnormal haemoglobin (HbS) polymerises, resulting in sickling of the red blood cells and blockage of the microcirculation.

(e) People of African or African—Caribbean origin are most often affected.

(f) Sickling occurs under low oxygen tensions and so sedation may cause a problem and may precipitate a crisis, hence should be avoided in general practice. General anaesthetics also have the potential to cause a sickling crisis and should only be given when absolutely necessary and following adequate preoperative assessment.

7.17 (a) What groups of analgesic drugs could you prescribe to a patient with dental pain? Give two side effects of each group?

(b) Given an example of a drug in each group.

(c) What are the contraindications of aspirin?

(d) How is paracetamol potentially lethal?

(e) What other properties does paracetamol have beside analgesia?

(f) Write a regimen for postoperative pain control for a fit and healthy patient whose lower wisdom tooth has been surgically extracted.

Answer 7.17

(a) Analgesics for dental pain and their side effects:
- NSAIDs — gastric ulceration, asthma attacks
- Aspirin (can be included in NSAIDs) — gastric ulceration, asthma attacks, allergic disease, Reye syndrome, hepatic impairment
- Opioids — respiratory depression, nausea, vomiting, constipation, dependence
- Paracetamol — liver damage, rashes, blood disorders (thrombocytopenia, leukopenia)

(b) Any one of the following:
- NSAIDs — ibuprofen, ketoprofen, diclofenac, mefenamic acid
- Aspirin
- Opioids — morphine, codeine, diamorphine, dihydrocodeine, codeine phosphate, fentanyl, papaveretum
- Paracetamol

(c) Contraindications of aspirin:
- Bleeding disorders
- Gastric or duodenal ulceration
- Patient under 12 years
- Asthma
- Pregnancy
- Allergy to aspirin

(d) It can cause liver toxicity.

(e) It is antipyretic.

(f) Postoperative pain control:
- Ibuprofen — 400 mg up to four times daily orally as required
- Paracetamol — 1 g up to four times daily orally as required
- Dihydrocodeine 30 mg up to four times daily orally as required
- Codeine phosphate 30 mg up to four times daily orally as required

7.18 (a) You are carrying out a dental extraction on a 70-year-old man in your practice. He pushes your hand away and tells you to stop leaning on his chest (which you are not doing). What is the likely diagnosis?

(b) What other symptoms may he be experiencing?

(c) How would you proceed in this situation?

(d) The pain continues and becomes more severe. He becomes pale, clammy and feels nauseous. What has happened?

(e) How would you proceed?

Answer 7.18

(a) Ischaemic chest pain (angina)

(b) The patient may also be experiencing:
- Central chest/retrosternal pain
- Band-like chest pain
- Pain radiating to the mandible/left arm

(c) Management of ischaemic chest pain:
1 Stop the procedure

2 Make the patient sit up

3 Administer sublingual GTN

4 Administer oxygen

(d) The ischaemic chest pain has progressed from angina (reversible) to myocardial infarction (irreversible).

(e) Management of myocardial infarction:
1 Call for help (ambulance).

2 Continue to give oxygen.

3 If you are able to establish intravenous access then do so (useful for opioid analgesics) but these are not readily available in dental practice. However should the patient proceed to cardiac arrest, intravenous access is useful.

4 Give analgesia nitrous oxide/oxygen mixture (50% oxygen).

7.19 (a) A pregnant woman needs to have dental treatment. When is the best time for carrying out the treatment and why?

(b) What are the potential problems with carrying out treatment at other times?

(c) What oral conditions may a pregnant woman present with?

(d) If a pregnant woman had a dental abscess, which of the following antibiotics can you prescribe for her?

- Penicillin

- Erythromycin

- Metronidazole

(e) If you needed to prescribe analgesics which ones could you prescribe and which ones would you avoid and why?

Answer 7.19

(a) Ideally major dental work should be delayed until after pregnancy. The best time to carry out treatment during pregnancy is probably the second trimester as it is important not to neglect dental health, eg pregnancy periodontitis.

(b) During the first trimester the fetus is most susceptible to teratogenic influences and abortion; 15% of pregnancies terminate in the first trimester. In the third trimester the risk of syncope is highest. Pressure on the inferior vena cava when the woman is supine leads to reduced venous return and hypotension. There is also the risk of pre-eclampsia.

(c) Oral conditions in pregnancy:
- Pyogenic granuloma/epulis

- Exacerbation of pre-existing gingivitis/periodontitis

- Pregnancy periodontitis

(d) In pregnancy the following can be prescribed:
- Penicillin

- Erythromycin

Note: drugs can have harmful effects on the fetus during pregnancy. During the first trimester there is the risk of teratogenesis (congenital malformation), and during the second and third trimesters, drugs may affect growth and functional development. Near term they may have adverse effects on labour or on the neonate after delivery. Metronidazole may be prescribed but high doses must be avoided.

(e) Paracetamol can be prescribed in pregnancy. It is not known to be harmful in pregnancy. Avoid opioid analgesics (eg codeine, tramadol, morphine). They can cause neonatal respiratory depression and withdrawal. NSAIDs can be associated with a risk of premature closure of the ductus arteriosus so they are contraindicated in the third trimester.

7.20 (a) What are the three characteristic features of asthma?

(b) Give three clinical features and signs that would make you suspect asthma in a patient.

(c) Name three groups of agents that are used in the treatment of asthma. How do they work?

(d) A 20-year-old patient with known asthma and concurrent coryza comes for dental treatment. During treatment he develops chest tightening and wheezing. How would you proceed?

Answer 7.20

(a) Characteristic features of asthma:
- Reversible airflow limitation
- Airway hyper-responsiveness to a range of stimuli
- Inflammation of the bronchi

(b) Any three of the following:
- Episodic wheeze or cough
- Shortness of breath
- Diurnal variation (symptoms worse at night and early morning)
- Expiratory polyphonic wheeze on auscultation
- Reduced chest expansion during asthma attack

(c) There is a stepwise approach in the management of a patient with asthma, which depends partly on their peak flow.
1. β_2-Adrenoreceptor agonists (eg salbutamol, terbutaline, salmeterol) — causes relaxation of bronchial smooth muscle and bronchial dilatation
2. Anti-cholinergic bronchodilator (eg ipratropium bromide) — causes bronchodilatation
3. Inhaled corticosteroids (eg beclomethasone, budesonide) — they are anti-inflammatory agents used as maintenance treatment
4. Sodium cromoglicate — prevents activation of inflammatory cells
5. Slow-release theophylline — relaxes smooth muscle

(d) Management of patient with known asthma and concurrent coryza:
1. Stop treatment
2. Make the patient sit upright
3. Follow ABC
4. Clear the patient's airway, use suction, if necessary. Remove all instruments. Check the patient has not inhaled any foreign body. If so remove by abdominal thrust (Heimlich's manoeuvre).
5. Give two puffs of salbutamol inhaler
6. Give oxygen 15 litres per minute
7. Call for help

7.21 (a) Select from the list below two conditions that diabetes mellitus may be secondary to:

- Corticosteroid treatment
- Chronic pancreatitis
- Obesity
- Insulin overproduction
- Insulin insufficiency
- Insulin resistance
- Insulin sensitivity

(b) Which of the above happens with regard to insulin?

(c) List four presenting features of diabetes mellitus.

(d) What dental manifestations may a diabetic patient present with?

(e) What is the most common diabetic emergency likely to present in general dental practice? What are the symptoms of this condition?

(f) If this condition occurs how would you manage it?

Answer 7.21

(a) Any two of the following:
- Corticosteroid treatment
- Chronic pancreatitis
- Obesity
- Insulin insufficiency
- Insulin resistance

(b)
- Insulin insufficiency
- Insulin resistance

(c) Any four of the following:
- Polyuria
- Polydipsia
- Weight loss
- Lethargy
- Recurrent infection

(d) Oral manifestations of diabetes:
- Chronic periodontal disease
- Increased susceptibility to infections/dental abscesses
- Xerostomia

(e) Hypoglycaemia. The patient may be irritable, disorientated, increasingly drowsy, excitable or aggressive. They may appear drunk, cold, sweaty and tachycardic.

(f) Check the blood glucose level to verify hypoglycaemia if you have the facility to do so otherwise presume hypoglycaemic episode. Then:
- If conscious give glucose orally in any form.
- If unconscious place in recovery position, give 1 mg glucagon intramuscularly, or obtain intravenous access if possible and administer 50 ml of 20–50% dextrose.

Note: in a diabetic patient it is safer to give glucose and not insulin if there are any concerns about the diagnosis.

7.22 (a) A new patient attends your practice with a medical history of epilepsy. What is epilepsy?

(b) Name two common types of epilepsy.

(c) Phenytoin is often given to patients to control their epilepsy. What are the dental implications of a patient taking phenytoin?

(d) Name two other drugs that are often used to control epilepsy.

(e) What do you understand by the term status epilepticus and how would you manage it in the dental surgery?

Answer 7.22

(a) It is a spontaneous intermittent abnormal electrical activity in a part of the brain that results in seizures.

(b) Any two of the following:
- Grand-mal epilepsy

- Petit-mal epilepsy

- Myoclonic

- Simple and complex focal seizures

(c) Patients given long-term phenytoin treatment may develop gingival hyperplasia.

(d) Any two of the following:
- Carbamazepine

- Sodium valproate

- Phenobarbital (phenobarbitone)

- Benzodiazepines

- Lamotrigine

(e) In status epilepticus fitting does not stop after 5 minutes or fits are rapidly repeated without intervening consciousness. Prolonged fitting is dangerous and may result in cerebral damage and hence prompt action is needed. An ambulance should be summoned as any patient with status epilepticus should go to hospital, even if they stop fitting and recover. Maintain the airway and administer oxygen, make sure that the patient is not likely to hurt themselves with equipment lying close to them. Administer 10 mg buccal midazolam while waiting for the ambulance. If needed the ambulance personnel will administer iv diazepam on arrival.

7.23 (a) What do you understand by the terms bacteraemia and septicaemia?

(b) Infective endocarditis may occur as a complication of dental treatment — what is infective endocarditis?

(c) Which organisms commonly cause infective endocarditis?

(d) Which patients are at risk of getting infective endocarditis from dental treatment?

(e) What precautions should be taken before carrying out subgingival scaling under local anaesthetic in a patient who has had previous endocarditis if they are allergic to penicillin?

Answer 7.23

(a) Bacteraemia means bacteria in the blood stream, usually at a low level and clinically not of consequence. Septicaemia is sepsis in the blood stream and is due to large numbers of organisms in the blood. Clinical features include rigours, fever and hypotension.

(b) Inflammation of the endocardium of the heart valves and endocardium around congenital defects of the heart from an infection.

(c) Bacteria most commonly cause infective endocarditis — usually *Streptococcus viridans*, *Streptococcus faecalis* (subacute infective endocarditis) and *Streptococcus pneumoniae*, *Staphylococcus aureus* and *Streptococcus pyogenes* (acute infective endocarditis); fungi, *Chlamydia* species and rickettsiae less commonly cause this condition.

(d) Theoretically those who have had previous endocarditis, those with prosthetic heart valves and those with surgically constructed systemic or pulmonary shunts or conduits are at risk of infective endocarditis from invasive dental treatment. However, they are also at risk of infective endocarditis from any bacteraemia and simple chewing may cause a bacteraemia. Because of this it is now thought that maintenance of a good standard of oral hygiene and health is more important than giving patients one-off doses of antibiotic when they undergo invasive dental treatment. Following the publication of new research at the AHA meeting in Chicago on 18 November, 2014, showing an increase in the incidence of infective endocarditis in the UK, NICE has launched an immediate review of CG64 on *Prophylaxis for Infective Endocarditis*.

(e) Some practitioners administer preoperative chlorhexidine mouthwashes.

7.24 (a) A 40-year-old man presents with a medical history of alcoholic liver disease and needs a dental extraction. What are your concerns and why?

(b) He is very anxious and requests sedation. Are there any contraindications?

(c) Which antibiotic could you safely prescribe this patient from the list below:

- Amoxicillin
- Flucloxacillin
- Erythromycin
- Tetracycline
- Doxycycline
- Metronidazole
- Clindamycin
- Cephalosporins

(d) The following is a list of commonly used drugs in dentistry. If you had a patient with renal failure how would this affect the prescription of the drugs? For each drug state whether you would prescribe it normally, reduce the dose or avoid it completely.

- Amoxicillin
- Metronidazole
- Tetracycline
- Miconazole
- Midazolam
- NSAIDs

Answer 7.24

(a) Alcoholic liver disease is a cause of liver cirrhosis. The liver is responsible for plasma proteins including clotting factors and for detoxification. The patient may have excessive bleeding following the extraction, so it is important to check for a history of abnormal bleeding.

(b) Due to reduced drug clearance, the use of sedatives should be avoided as coma is a risk.

(c) Amoxicillin, flucloxacillin, cephalosporins

(d) Dose alterations in renal failure:
  - Amoxicillin — reduce dose
  - Metronidazole — prescribe normally
  - Tetracycline — avoid
  - Miconazole — reduce dose
  - Midazolam — reduce dose
  - NSAIDs — avoid

7.25   Look at the full blood count (FBC) results and choose from the list below the condition the patient may have, the appearance on the blood film and the possible causes:

- Macrocytic anaemia
- Microcytic anaemia
- Hypochromic anaemia
- Normocytic anaemia
- Iron deficiency
- Vitamin B_{12} deficiency
- Folate deficiency
- Anaemia of chronic disease
- Thalassaemia
- Blood loss
- Alcoholism

(a) Full blood count:

		Reference interval
Haemoglobin (Hb)	108 g/l	135—180 g/l (female), 115—160 g/l (male)
Packed cell volume (PCV)	0.33 l/l	0.37—0.47 l/l (female), 0.4—0.54 l/l (male)
Mean corpuscular volume (MCV)	72 fl	76—79 fl
Mean corpuscular haemoglobin (MCH)	25 pg	27—32 pg
Mean corpuscular haemoglobin concentration (MCHC)	280 g/l	300—360 g/l
White cell count (WCC)	6.6×10^9/l	$4.0—11 \times 10^9$/l
Platelets	207×10^9/l	$150—400 \times 10^9$/l

(b) Full blood count:

		Reference interval
Haemoglobin (Hb)	98 g/l	135—180 g/l (female), 115—160 g/l (male)
Packed cell volume (PCV)	0.6 l/l	0.37—0.47 l/l (female), 0.4—0.54 l/l (male)
Mean corpuscular volume (MCV)	84 fl	76—79 fl
Mean corpuscular haemoglobin (MCH)	28 pg	27—32 pg
Mean corpuscular haemoglobin concentration (MCHC)	320 g/l	300—360 g/l
White cell count (WCC)	8.2×10^9/l	$4.0—11 \times 10^9$/l
Platelets	255×10^9/l	$150—400 \times 10^9$/l

(c) List five signs and symptoms of anaemia (not including intraoral ones).

Answer 7.25

(a) FBC shows microcytic hypochromic anaemia:
   - Microcytic anaemia
   - Hypochromic anaemia
   - Iron deficiency
   - Thalassaemia
   - Blood loss

(b) FBC shows macrocytic anaemia consistent with:
   - Vitamin B_{12} deficiency
   - Folate deficiency
   - Alcoholism

(c) The signs depend on the severity of the anaemia. They range from lethargy, pallor and weakness to dizziness, tinnitus, vertigo, headache and dyspnoea (shortness of breath) on exertion, tachycardia, palpitations, angina, cardiac failure and gastrointestinal disturbances.

7.26 Give two features seen in each of the syndromes listed below.

Syndrome	Features
Apert	
Crouzon	
Treacher Collins	
Albright	
Pierre—Robin	
Goldenhar	
Van der Woude	
Gardener	
Down	
Gorlin—Goltz	
Ramsay—Hunt	
Peutz—Jeghers	

Answer 7.26

Any two of the features given in the table below:

Syndrome	Features
Apert	Craniosynostosis (premature closure of sutures of skull), fused fingers and toes, can be associated with cleft palate, maxillary hypoplasia
Crouzon	Shallow orbits, proptosis, conductive hearing loss, may have small maxilla
Treacher Collins	Underdeveloped or absent cheekbone and abnormal shape of the eyes, malformed or absent ears, micrognathia
Albright	Café-au-lait patches, polyostotic fibrous dysplasia, endocrine dysfunction, precocious puberty
Pierre—Robin	Prominent tongue, micrognathia, cleft palate
Goldenhar	Bilateral craniofacial microsomia, epibulbar dermoids, vertebral anomalies
Van der Woude	Lower lip pits, cleft lip
Gardener	Multiple osteomas, intestinal polyps, cysts, skin fibromas
Down	Flattened nasal bridge, upward sloping palpebral fissures, midface retrusion, class III malocclusion, macroglossia, delayed tooth eruption, heart defects, atlantoaxial subluxation
Gorlin—Goltz	Basal cell carcinomas, keratocysts, parietal bossing, bifid ribs, calcification of the falx cerebri
Ramsay—Hunt	Lower motor neurone facial palsy, vesicles, herpes zoster of the geniculate ganglion
Peutz—Jeghers	Intestinal polyps, perioral pigmentation

7.27 (a) A new patient has collapsed in your waiting room. Outline your initial management of the situation.

(b) If he is unresponsive how will you proceed?

(c) If you need to do cardiopulmonary resuscitation what ratio of chest compressions to breaths will you use?

(d) How many chest compressions are you aiming to complete per minute?

(e) Where will you place your hands to do the compressions?

(f) By how much are you attempting to compress the chest?

(g) How long should you take over your rescue breaths?

(h) How long are you going to continue resuscitating for?

Answer 7.27

(a) Initial management:

    1 Check the area is safe.

    2 Try to arouse the patient by shaking and shouting to him in both ears.

    3 If there is no response shout for help and proceed to resuscitation.

(b) If the patient is unresponsive:

    1 Shout for help.

    2 Follow ABC resuscitation guidelines.

    3 Check airway and clear it and open it if necessary.

    4 Check breathing — look, listen and feel for no more than 10 seconds.

    5 If there are no signs of breathing go for help and call ambulance (or get someone else to go if you are not alone).

    6 Give 30 chest compressions.

    7 Give 2 rescue breaths.

    8 Give 30 chest compressions, etc.

(c) 30 compressions to 2 breaths

(d) 100–120 chest compressions per minute

(e) In the centre of the chest

(f) 5–6 cm in an adult per compression

(g) 1 second for each breath

(h) Until help comes or you become exhausted or the patient recovers (Note: this is based on the Resuscitation Council UK Guidelines 2010)

7.28   The following are drugs that you may have in your emergency box. In which conditions and how you would use them? How you would recognise each condition?

- Glyceryl trinitrate
- Adrenaline/epinephrine
- Salbutamol
- Aspirin

Answer 7.28

- Glyceryl trinitrate — sublingual spray or tablet, used in angina. Angina is acute chest pain due to myocardial ischaemia. Patients feel central crushing chest pain which may radiate down their left arm or a band-like chest pain. There may also be shortness of breath.

- Adrenaline/epinephrine — intramuscularly 0.5 ml of 1:1000. Given in anaphylaxis, which usually occurs following administration of a drug. Patients have facial flushing with itching or tingling. There may be facial oedema and lip swelling and urticaria. There is bronchospasm (wheezing) and hypotension. If not treated there will be loss of consciousness and cardiac arrest.

- Salbutamol — two puffs from inhaler in asthma. If there is no response use a salbutamol nebuliser. Asthmatic patients experience breathlessness, wheeze on expiration and inability to talk. They will use their accessory muscles of respiration in an attempt to breathe. Tachycardia and cyanosis may also occur.

- Aspirin — 300 mg oral in myocardial infarction. Patients have a central crushing chest pain, which does not respond to glyceryl trinitrate. There may be vomiting, sweating, pallor, cold clammy skin and shortness of breath and the patient may progress to loss of consciousness.

7.29 (a) What is shock?

(b) Septic and cardiogenic are two different types of shock. Name two other types of shock.

(c) Fill in the blanks in the table about the features of a particular type of shock.

Type of shock	Associated features	Peripheral temperature	Central venous pressure
	Dehydrated/ blood loss		Reduced

Note: peripheral temperature may be increased, decreased or stay the same.

(d) What do you understand by the term Addisonian crisis?

(e) If this occurs in the dental surgery how should it be managed?

Answer 7.29

(a) Shock is acute circulatory failure leading to inadequate tissue perfusion and end-organ injury or inadequate tissue oxygenation/organ perfusion.

(b) Any two of the following:
- Hypovolaemic
- Anaphylactic
- Neurogenic

(c)

Type of shock	Associated features	Peripheral temperature	Central venous pressure
Hypovolaemic	Dehydrated/ blood loss	Decreased	Reduced

(d) In Addison's disease there is a failure of secretion of cortisol and aldosterone and patients are treated with steroids. In times of stress such as infections, surgery or anaesthesia the body cannot respond due to the inadequate corticosteroid production. This results in a rapid fall in blood pressure, which leads to circulatory collapse and shock. This is known as an addisonian crisis.

(e) Management of addisonian crisis:
1 Lie the patient flat and raise their legs

2 Call for help (ambulance)

3 Oxygen.

4 Intravenous fluids and hydrocortisone sodium succinate 100–200 mg iv may be administered but only if you are familiar with their use.

8
General Dentistry

8.1   One of the nine core ethical principles to which the General Dental Council states registered dental professionals must adhere is to raise concerns if patients are at risk.

(a) What are the other eight principles?

(b) What issues may patients be at risk of that you would need to report or raise?

(c) In what instance(s) would it be inappropriate to raise concerns?

(d) If you are the practice manager and a member of the dental team has raised a concern with you, what steps must you take and how would you manage the situation?

Answer 8.1

(a)

- Put patient's interests first
- Communicate effectively with patients
- Obtain valid consent
- Maintain and protect patient information
- Have a clear and effective complaints procedure
- Work with colleagues in a way that is in patient's best interest
- Maintain, develop and work within your professional knowledge and skills
- Make sure that your personal behaviour maintains patient confidence in you and the dental profession

(b)

- The health, behaviour or professional performance of a colleague
- Being asked to do something that you feel conflicts with your duty to put patients' interests first
- The environment in which treatment is carried out

(c) It is never inappropriate to raise concerns. You must raise concerns even if you are not in a position to control or influence your working environment, or if you feel that raising concerns may be disloyal to your colleagues or bosses. Raising concerns overrides any personal and professional loyalties.

(d) It is important to take every concern seriously and maintain confidentiality while dealing with the concern. Your investigation should be carried out promptly and the individual should be kept informed of the progress of the investigation and any action taken. You must act in an unbiased manner and any action taken to solve the problem must be monitored.

8.2 (a) What factors would you take into account in order to assess an individual's caries risk?

(b) How frequently should you take bitewing radiographs for adult patients who fall into the high- and low-caries risk categories?

(c) What is the radiation dose from a bitewing radiograph?

Answer 8.2

(a) To assess caries risk various factors should be taken into account:

Social history:

- Social/economic status: the caries rate is known to be higher in those from deprived backgrounds

- Caries rate of siblings

- Attendance record: poor attendees tend to have poorer oral health

- Low dental knowledge and expectations

Medical history:

- Long-term usage of sugar-containing medications

- Medical conditions that cause xerostomia

- Disabilities that make maintaining oral hygiene difficult

Dietary habits:

- Frequent and high sugar intake

Fluoride usage:

- Live in an area with or without water fluoridation

- Use of fluoride toothpaste and supplements

Oral hygiene:

- Ineffective cleaning, plaque-retentive factors

Saliva:

- Low flow rate/xerostomia

- High counts of *Streptococcus mutans* and lactobacilli

Clinical appearance:

- Evidence of new carious lesions

- Missing teeth from extractions

- Smooth surface caries

- Heavily restored dentition

- No evidence of fissure sealants

- Wears an appliance that will make maintaining oral health more difficult

(b) According to the *FGDP Selection Criteria for GDPs* (3rd edition), adults who are in the low-caries risk category should have posterior bitewing radiographs at 2-yearly intervals, but, if there is evidence of continuing low-caries risk, the interval may be extended. For those at a high risk of caries, the bitewings should be taken at 6-monthly intervals until no new or active lesions are apparent.

(c) The effective dose from a bitewing radiograph is between 0.3 and 21.6 mSv.

8.3 (a) You are a general dental practitioner in practice. One of your patients has tonsillar carcinoma and is due to have radiotherapy as part of his treatment regimen. What are the side effects of radiotherapy on the oral environment?

(b) Following the radiotherapy what is the role of the general dental practitioner in maintaining oral health?

Answer 8.3

(a) The oral side effects of radiotherapy can be divided into immediate and late. They are dose related and, if the patient receives over 60 Gy, then they are significant.

Immediate side effects include:

- Mucositis which often occurs after about 2–3 weeks of treatment and presents as widespread erythema, bleeding, ulceration and pain. These usually subside after the radiotherapy is completed.

- Xerostomia which may occur after only a week of radiotherapy. The extent of the dryness will depend on the fields irradiated; if both parotid glands are irradiated then it is severe.

- Alteration in taste and difficulty swallowing

- Weight loss

Late or long-term side effects include:

- Xerostomia continues after the radiotherapy treatment and is responsible for most of the long-term conditions associated with radiotherapy treatment.

- Radiation-associated caries may occur due to the reduced salivary flow rate, and is made worse if patients have a highly cariogenic diet.

- Candida infections may occur due to the reduced salivary flow rate.

- Osteoradionecrosis may occur if there is trauma to the jaws in an irradiated field, the most common trauma being tooth extraction, although trauma from dentures may cause it. It is a painful and debilitating condition that is very difficult to treat; for this reason prevention is better than cure. All patients who are due to have radiotherapy must have a dental assessment before the treatment and removal of any teeth of dubious prognosis should occur well in advance of the start of the radiotherapy, to allow the sockets time to heal.

- Trismus may occur due to fibrosis caused by the radiotherapy; this often occurs if the muscles of mastication are in the radiation field, especially the medial pterygoid (note that it may also occur as a result of surgery to treat cancer).

- Weight loss may occur due to difficulties eating as a result of soreness or dryness. Loss of taste and difficulty swallowing may also hamper eating, leading to weight loss.

(b) The patient will receive support form the oncological team and restorative dentist but will also need the input of their own general dental practitioner:
  - Maintenance

  - Frequent check-ups

  - Check for any new pathology

It is imperative that patients maintain a good standard of oral hygiene (both during and after the treatment). The general dental practitioner will need to play an active role overseeing this, whether it be by brushing or by use of chlorhexidine gluconate mouthwashes. The use of sponges may be needed if cleaning becomes too painful.

Dietary advice
  - Advice re oral dryness — avoid sucking sugary sweets to stimulate salivary flow

  - Use salivary substitutes

  - Fluoride and chlorhexidine regimens

  - Referral for any dental extractions

8.4 (a) What is evidence-based dentistry?

(b) What are the levels of evidence?

(c) Which is the strongest evidence?

(d) What are the levels of recommendation?

Answer 8.4

(a) Evidence-based dentistry is the integration of current scientific evidence with clinical expertise and patient values. It is the use of current scientific evidence to guide decision-making in dentistry.

(b) The following is the hierarchy of evidence for quantitative questions:
- Level I: evidence from a systematic review of all the relevant randomised controlled trials (RCTs), or evidence-based clinical practice guidelines, based on systematic reviews of RCTs

- Level II: evidence obtained from at least one well-designed RCT

- Level III: evidence obtained from well-designed controlled trials without randomisation; quasi-experimental

- Level IV: evidence from well-designed case–control and cohort studies

- Level V: evidence from systematic reviews of descriptive and qualitative studies

- Level VI: evidence from a single descriptive or qualitative study

- Level VII: evidence from the opinion of authorities and/or reports of expert committees

(c) The strongest evidence is a level I systematic review of all relevant RCTs or evidence-based clinical practice guidelines based on systematic reviews of RCTs.

(d) The following are the levels of recommendation:
- Level A: good scientific evidence suggests that the benefits of the clinical service substantially outweigh the potential risks.

- Level B: at least fair scientific evidence suggests that the benefits of the clinical service outweigh the potential risks.

- Level C: at least fair scientific evidence suggests that there are benefits provided by the clinical service, but the balance between benefits and risks are too close to make general recommendations.

- Level D: at least fair scientific evidence suggests that the risks of the clinical service outweigh potential benefits.

- Level E: scientific evidence is lacking, of poor quality or conflicting, such that the risk-versus-benefit balance cannot be assessed.

8.5 (a) When assessing an unwell patient we follow the ABCDE approach. What does each of these letters stand for?

(b) Briefly describe how you would assess the C, D and E components in an unwell patient in your dental practice.

Answer 8.5

(a) Airway, Breathing, Circulation, Disability, Exposure

(b) C Circulation

- As you approach the assessment in a systematic manner going from A to B to C you will already have all the information from the A and B assessment prior to starting the C assessment.

- Take the radial pulse of the patient and assess rate and rhythm. If you are familiar with taking a carotid pulse then do so, but do not attempt it if you are not familiar with the method.

- Take the blood pressure.

- Look at the colour of the patient's hands and fingers for any signs of mottling, pallor or cyanosis.

- Assess the capillary refill time by pressing on a finger tip held at the level of the heart for 5 seconds, which will cause it to blanch. The normal colour should return in 2 seconds due to capillary refill, longer than this implies a poor peripheral circulation. When doing this you will also be able to assess the warmth of the hand, which again if very cold may imply poor peripheral circulation.

- Also determine whether the patient has any chest pain.

D Disability

- Using the AVPU system, assess the conscious level of the patient. A = alert, V = responds to vocal stimuli, P = responds to pain and U = unresponsive.

- Check the blood glucose level if you have the appropriate equipment.

- Examine the eyes and assess the size of both of the pupils and whether they react equally to light.

- Check which drugs/medicines the patient usually takes.

E Exposure

- This means looking at the patient's body to see if there is a clue as to the cause of the problem, eg bleeding or a rash etc. However, the patient must be kept warm and you must respect their dignity.

For further information on the ABCDE approach, see www.resus.org.uk.

8.6 (a) What are the indications for professionally applied topical fluorides (PATFs)?

(b) Fluoride varnishes are a commonly used type of professionally applied topical fluoride. What other types are available?

(c) What is the concentration of fluoride in commonly available fluoride varnishes?

(d) What are the advantages of fluoride varnishes over other PATF preparations?

Answer 8.6

(a) PATFs are appropriate for patients who have been identified as having a high risk of dental caries including:

- Those who are at high risk of caries on smooth surfaces and root surfaces

- Those with decreased salivary flow rates

- Those undergoing radiotherapy of the head and neck

- Those undergoing orthodontic treatment

- Children, who should have their permanent molars sealed but for whatever reason they cannot be sealed

(b)

- Fluoride gel

- Fluoride foam

- Fluoride rinses

(c) The amount varies greatly depending on the preparation. Some common ones are listed below:

- Duraphat (Colgate Oral Pharmaceuticals): concentration 26 000 ppm (2.2% F⁻)

- Biofluorid 12 (VOCO Chemi GmbH): concentration 56 300 ppm

- Fluor Protector (Ivoclar-Viviadent): concentration 7000 ppm

- Fluor Protector (Ivoclar-Viviadent): concentration 1000 ppm (0.1% F⁻)

(d)

- Easy to apply, no special trays or equipment needed.

- The varnish is applied and then sets, so no drying is needed and the patient can close their mouth immediately following treatment, whereas when using a gel it is necessary to leave it on for 4 minutes to gain the optimal fluoride uptake.

- If necessary it can be targeted to specific areas whereas with a gel this is not so easy.

- It can be carried out on young children who do not tolerate the trays.

- Less likelihood of excessive ingestion of fluoride, which may occur if trays of gel are overfilled.

8.7 (a) What do you understand by the term infection control with respect to the dental surgery?

(b) What are the three main routes by which infection be transmitted in a dental practice? For each of the routes please give an example of a pathogen that may be transmitted via this route.

(c) Describe the differences, and the reasons behind the differences, in infection control procedures which you would employ in dental practice when treating

- A patient with diagnosed HIV

- A patient with no known blood-borne diseases

(d) Hand hygiene is an important part of an overall infection control routine. When should hand hygiene be practised in dentistry?

(e) What areas and items of equipment in the vicinity of a dental chair need to be cleaned between each patient?

Answer 8.7

(a) A series of measures undertaken to prevent the route of transmission of pathogens within the dental surgery.

(b) Transmission via direct or indirect contact:
- Eg viruses — herpes, varicella-zoster, Epstein—Barr, hepatitis, respiratory syncytial

- Eg bacteria — meticillin-resistant *Staphylococcus aureus* (MRSA)

Parenteral transmission via the blood stream
- Viruses — hepatitis B, hepatitis D, human immunodeficiency virus (HIV)

Transmission via airborne and respiratory secretions
- Bacteria — tuberculosis

- Viruses — influenza, severe acute respiratory syndrome (SARS), coronavirus

(c) You would treat each patient in exactly the same manner and employ universal precautions. The reasoning is that universal precautions should be sufficient to stop the transmission of any infectious agent and should be employed with all patients as you may not know which of your patients have a blood-borne disease.

(d) Hand hygiene should be carried out:
- At the beginning and end of each treatment session

- Before donning personal protective equipment (PPE) and after removing PPE

- Following the washing of dental instruments

- Before contact with instruments that have been steam-sterilised (whether or not these instruments are wrapped)

- Following cleaning or maintaining decontamination devices used on dental instruments

- Following the completion of decontamination work.

These are stipulations published by the Department of Health in the document *Decontamination. Health Technical Memorandum 01—05: Decontamination in primary care dental practices* (2009).

(e) *Decontamination. Health Technical Memorandum 01–05: Decontamination in primary care dental practices* states that the following items within a dental surgery should be cleaned between patients:
- Dental chairs
- Local work surfaces
- Curing lamps
- Inspection lights and handles
- Hand controls including replacement of covers
- Trolleys/delivery units
- Spittoons
- Aspirators
- X-ray units

8.8 (a) What do you understand by the term decontamination in relation to primary care dental practice?

(b) While working in a dental surgery you will produce waste that is categorised as hazardous due to it being infectious. However, the term hazardous waste encompasses other items as well. What do you understand by the term hazardous waste? Please give some examples.

(c) Why are some dental practices required to register as a hazardous waste producer, but some are not?

(d) What are the responsibilities of the registered manager of the practice with regard to waste?

Answer 8.8

(a) Decontamination is the process by which reusable items are rendered safe for further use and for staff to handle. Decontamination is required to minimise the risk of cross-infection between patients and between patients and staff.

The Department of Health document *Decontamination. Health Technical Memorandum 01–05: Decontamination in primary care dental practices* published in 2009 contains guidance on decontamination in primary care dental practice.

(b) Hazardous waste has one or more properties that are harmful to a person's health or the environment. It includes explosive, highly flammable, carcinogenic, oxidising, irritant, infectious, teratogenic, mutagenic, and harmful waste and toxic gases.

Examples of hazardous waste are:
- Dental amalgam

- Photographic fixer

- Photographic developer

- Clinical waste, eg dressings contaminated with body fluids, personal protective equipment and swabs, and other waste that may present a risk of infection

(c) All dental practices that produce 500 kg or more of hazardous waste in any 12-month period need to register their premises annually, as decreed by the Hazardous Waste (Amendment) Regulations 2009.

If the practice produces less than 500 kg in any 12-month period, it is exempt.

(d) It is the responsibility of the registered manager of the practice to ensure that waste is:
- Correctly segregated (there is a colour-coded waste segregation and packaging system that aids standardised identification of waste)

- Stored safely and securely away from areas of public access within the premises

- Packaged appropriately for transport

- Described accurately and fully on the accompanying documentation when removed

- Transferred to an authorised person for transport to an authorised waste site

- Appropriately registered, with necessary records and returns at premises

They also need to ensure that staff are trained and aware of the waste procedures.

8.9 (a) Different types of autoclave are available for use in dental practices: type N, type B and type S. What are the differences between them?

(b) How would you test your autoclave in general practice and how would you record such tests?

(c) How would you store instruments that had been sterilised in a dental practice?

(d) Instruments should be used within a certain time frame. What are the maximum times instruments can be stored following autoclaving in a
  - Type N steriliser?
  - Type B steriliser?

Answer 8.9

(a)

- Type N — designed for solid non-wrapped instruments as the air inside them is removed by passive displacement with steam.

- Type B — designed for hollow, air retentive and packaged loads, as they have a vacuum stage

- Type S — designed for specific loads as defined by the manufacturer. They are not commonly used in general dental practice.

(b) Testing is important to ensure that the autoclave is performing as expected. Each autoclave should have a log book into which the various details are entered and saved. These include:
   - Routine tests carried out

   - Maintenance carried out

   - Faults that have occurred

   - Validation and any modifications carried out

   Basic daily testing should occur prior to use each day but a schedule for further testing (in accordance with the manufacturer's guidelines) should also be planned and recorded in the log book.

   Daily testing for all small sterilisers would include an automatic control test in accordance with manufacturer's guidelines, and for vacuum-type (type B) autoclaves, a steam penetration test (Helix or Bowie–Dick test).

(c) All sterilised instruments must be protected to ensure that they do not become contaminated prior to use. To do this they must be protected against pathogens, and hence a barrier(s) must be maintained between the instruments and the practice environment. They should also be stored in a dry area and protected against excessive heat.

   Information regarding regulations relating to infection control and sterilisation in general practice can be found in the Department of Health document *Decontamination. Health Technical Memorandum 01–05: Decontamination in primary care dental practices* (2009).

(d) The maximum storage time is 21 days for a type N steriliser and 60 days for a type B steriliser.

8.10 (a) Define what is meant by conscious sedation.

(b) Conscious sedation is commonly administered by the iv route but can be given via alternative routes. Name three routes for administering conscious sedation and the most commonly used drug for each route.

(c) How would you monitor a patient to whom you had administered an iv drug to create a state of conscious sedation?

(d) Who should carry out these checks?

(e) What equipment is needed to carry out these checks?

(f) Would this differ if you were administering conscious sedation via an inhalational method?

Answer 8.10

(a) Conscious sedation is defined as: 'A technique in which the use of a drug or drugs produces a state of depression of the central nervous system enabling treatment to be carried out, but during which verbal contact with the patient is maintained throughout the period of sedation. The drugs and techniques used to provide conscious sedation for dental treatment should carry a margin of safety wide enough to render loss of consciousness unlikely.'

Source: *Conscious sedation in the provision of dental care, a report of an Expert Group on Sedation for Dentistry, Standing Dental Advisory Committee* (Department of Health, 2003, www.dh.gov.uk).

(b)

- Inhalational — nitrous oxide and oxygen with a minimum of 30% oxygen

- Oral — midazolam or other benzodiazepine

- Intranasal — midazolam or other benzodiazepine

(c) Perform careful clinical monitoring that includes:
- Talking to the patient to assess their level of responsiveness

- Looking at their colour

- Ensuring their airway is clear

- Monitoring their breathing and their oxygen saturation

- Monitoring their pulse

- Monitoring their blood pressure

(d) It is essential that all members of the clinical team are capable of carrying out these checks, but it is essential that each member of the team knows what their exact role is when treating and monitoring a patient.

(e) A pulse oximeter and blood pressure-recording device (manual or electronic)

(f) Yes, it is accepted that clinical monitoring of the patient without additional electronic devices is adequate.

8.11 (a) What are the indications for conscious sedation in dentistry?

(b) What instructions would you give a patient to prepare them for an appointment when iv conscious sedation is to be carried out?

(c) Midazolam is a commonly used drug for iv sedation. What is its mode of action?

(d) Describe how you would administer midazolam to a patient requiring iv sedation.

(e) There is a reversal agent that may be used in emergency situations. What is this drug and how would you administer it?

Answer 8.11

(a)

- To treat patients who are anxious, or have a phobia of dental treatment

- To treat patients with a gag reflex that makes dental treatment difficult

- To treat patients who have movement disorders, or those with a physical and/or mental disorder who are otherwise unlikely to tolerate dental treatment

- To treat patients who are not phobic but are having an unpleasant procedure such as third molar surgery or a prolonged procedure

- To avoid a patient having a general anaesthetic for a procedure

- As part of a programme to introduce them to treatment under local anaesthesia

(b)

- To bring an escort (a responsible adult) to take them from the surgery, after the procedure, to a suitable setting. The escort must not bring children with them who would also need caring for.

- To only take light food and clear, non-alcoholic liquids prior to an appointment and not to have a big meal before they arrive (note: local policies differ; some state that the patient must starve for 6 hours as they would for general anaesthesia, however, the Department of Health guidelines state that fasting is not required).

- To take any medication as usual before attending.

- Inform them of the need to: have time off work afterwards and not drive, cycle or operate machinery or being the sole carer for children or relatives, or signing any legally binding documents for 24 hours.

Any postoperative instructions relative to the procedure carried out should be given to the escort verbally and a written copy should also be given when the procedure is completed and the patient is ready for discharge, after treatment.

The patient should also have all the relevant information regarding the procedure they were due to have carried out in order for them to give informed consent and sign a written consent form.

(c) Midazolam is a benzodiazepine drug and acts on benzodiazepine receptors in the central nervous system. This causes blockage of the γ-aminobutyric acid (GABA) receptors which causes an increase in length of time for repolarisation to occur after a neuron has been depolarised. This has the effect of reducing the number of stimuli that reach the higher centres and results in sedation.

(d) Midazolam is given as a solution of 1 mg in 1 ml, usually from a 10-ml vial. There is no exact amount to give a patient and the drug is titrated against the patient's response. Initially 2 mg is administered slowly. There is then a pause (at least 90 seconds) while the effect of that dose on the patient is assessed. In some cases that may be all that is required to reach an acceptable level of sedation. If not then a further increment of 1 mg is administered and the reaction judged. Further increments can be administered until an ideal level of sedation is reached, pausing for 30 seconds between increments to assess the effect of that increment.

(e) Flumazenil is administered intravenously. It is supplied as 100 mg/ml in a 5-ml ampoule, and usually 200 mg (2 ml) are administered over 15 seconds and then the response assessed and further 100-mg increments may be given at 60-second intervals if needed.

8.12 (a) What do you understand by the terms mean, mode and median?

(b) Using the DMF scores of 15 patients given below, work out the mean, mode and median of the results.

Patient	DMF score
1	2
2	3
3	7
4	0
5	1
6	8
7	3
8	11
9	6
10	3
11	7
12	0
13	10
14	3
15	4

(c) What does the term standard deviation (SD) describe and what is the SD for this group of DMF scores?

(d) What is the difference between specificity and sensitivity?

(e) Here are the results of some vitality tests of 50 upper first permanent molars using a new type of pulp tester. What is the sensitivity and specificity of this new test?

	True vital teeth	True non-vital teeth
Vital with pulp tester	28	2
Non-vital with pulp tester	5	15

(f) How does this differ from the positive predictive value, and what would the positive predictive value be in this case?

Answer 8.12

(a) In a series of measurements mean is the average measurement, mode is the most frequently observed measurement and median is the mid-most measurement.

(b)
- Mean = 4.53
- Mode = 3
- Median = 3

(c) The standard deviation is a measure of the variability of the results, so in this case it is how much the DMF scores vary from the mean DMF score of 4.53. To calculate the SD each of the differences is taken and squared and then the sum of the squared values is divided by $(n - 1)$ where n is the size of the sample. So in this case:

SD = square root of the sum of $(x - \text{mean } x)^2/n - 1$ = 3.46.

(d) Sensitivity is the proportion of cases that are recorded as having a condition and that really do have the condition. It can be expressed as the following formula:

Sensitivity = true positives/true positives + false negative

Specificity is the proportion of cases that are recorded as not having a condition and that actually do not have the condition, that is they are true negatives. It can be expressed as the following formula:

Specificity = true negatives/true negatives + false positives

(e) It is often easier to work out sensitivity and specificity using a table as shown below:

	Vital teeth	Non-vital teeth	
Vital with pulp tester	28 = true positive	2 = false positive	Positive predictive value = true positive/true positive and false positive 28/28 + 2 = 93%
Non-vital with pulp tester	5 = false negative	15 = true negative	
	Sensitivity = true positive/true positives + false negatives 28/28 + 5 = 85%	Specificity = true negative/true negative + false positive 15/15 + 2 = 88%	

(f) Positive predictive value means the proportion of cases who really do have the condition and tested positive out of those who tested positive for a condition.

8.13 (a) Patients may present with a pronounced gag reflex, which is sometimes anxiety induced. What other factors may cause a patient to have a pronounced gag reflex?

(b) What do you understand the term anxiety, and how does it differ from fear and phobia?

(c) What strategies may be used to aid gagging reduction so that dental treatment can be carried out more comfortably?

Answer 8.13

(a) The stimulus for gagging can be somatic, which means that touching a trigger area stimulates that individual to gag and the trigger areas differ from individual to individual. Or the stimulus may be psychogenic, which means there does not have to be direct physical contact with a trigger area to precipitate gagging. However, it is unlikely to be a single aetiological factor that causes a pronounced gag reflex in most patients. Some factors that may contribute to a patient having a pronounced gag reflex are:

- Anatomical — alteration in soft palate and posterior tongue anatomy

- Medical — eg nasal obstruction, heavy smoking, post-nasal drip, sinusitis, diaphragmatic hernia, motor neuron disease, and following head trauma (note: in some patients with motor neuron disease the gag reflex is absent)

- Psychological — fear, anxiety and dental phobia

- Iatrogenic — this is probably not abnormal but a response to poorly positioned instruments and materials by dental personnel!

(b)

- Anxiety is a subjective state defined as an unpleasant feeling of apprehension or impending danger in the presence of a real or perceived stimulus that the individual has learned to associate with a threat to well-being. It is often out of proportion to the real threat and is often associated with somatic symptoms such as sweating, tremors, palpitations, nausea, hyperventilation, etc.

- Fear is an appropriate defensive response to a real threat. It differs from anxiety as the response is brief and the danger external and definable. The associated somatic feelings stop when the danger stops.

- Phobia is an irrational fear of a situation or object. Reaction to the stimulus is greatly exaggerated with respect to the reality of the threat. It is not under voluntary control and the usual coping strategy is avoidance of the situation or object.

(c)

- Relaxation, distraction, desensitisation techniques

- Psychological and behavioural therapies

- Pharmacological agents — conscious sedation with nitrous oxide or with iv midazolam, or administration of local anaesthetic in the posterior maxilla prior to impression taking

- Complementary therapies, acupuncture, acupressure, transcutaneous nerve stimulation (TENS) and hypnosis

- Other practical techniques — eg closed mouth inferior alveolar nerve blocks, use of sectional impression trays, use of rubber dam to prevent liquid going down the back of the throat

8.14 (a) What does CQC stand for and what is its remit?

(b) What is the difference between CQC and the GDC?

(a) CQC stands for the Care Quality Commission. CQC is the health and social care regulator for England since April 2011. Their aim is to ensure better care for everyone in hospital, in a care home, at home and in the primary dental care sector.

All providers of the primary dental care services need to be registered and meet the essential standards of quality and safety. The CQC:

- Monitors how providers comply with the standards

- Gathers information and visits practices when needed

- Has enforcement power, eg it can issue fines and public warnings if services drop below the essential standards

- Can even close a service down if necessary if a patient's rights or safety are at risk

- Acts to protect patients whose rights are restricted under the Mental Health Act

- Promotes improvement in services

- Conducts regular reviews of how well those who arrange and provide services locally are performing

- Carries out special reviews of particular types of services and pathways of care, or undertakes investigations in areas where it has concerns about quality

The CQC also seeks the views of people who use the services and provides information to the public about the quality of their local care services. This, in turn, helps providers and commissioners of services to learn from each other about what works best and where improvement is needed, and helps to shape national policy.

(b) The CQC and the General Dental Council (GDC) both have major roles in regulating dentistry. CQC is the statutory system regulator of providers of regulated activities in England, and GDC is the statutory professional regulator of dentists and dental clinical professionals throughout the UK.

8.15 What do the following commonly used abbreviations stand for?

- IOTN
- OM radiograph
- BPE
- dmfs
- DMFT
- INR
- ESR
- CPITN
- MMPA
- MTA

Answer 8.15

- IOTN — index of treatment need
- OM radiograph — occipitomental radiograph
- BPE — basic periodontal examination
- dmfs — decayed missing and filled tooth surfaces of deciduous teeth
- DMFT — decayed missing and filled teeth in permanent teeth
- INR — international normalised ratio (used for measuring the efficacy of and monitoring anticoagulant treatment)
- ESR — erythrocyte sedimentation rate
- CPITN — community periodontal index of treatment need
- MMPA — maxillary–mandibular planes angle
- MTA — mineral trioxide aggregate

8.16 (a) Dental practices should have a written infection control protocol. List six elements that should be included in this document.

(b) How can clinical staff protect themselves from the risk of infection from patients?

(c) What do you understand by the term universal precautions?

(d) Name one condition for which additional measures are used.

Answer 8.16

(a) Any six of the following:
- Patient evaluation

- Personal protection

- Staff training in infection control measures

- Instrument management with respect to cleaning, sterilisation and storage

- Disinfection

- Disposable instruments

- Waste disposal

- Laboratory asepsis

(b) Protection against cross-infection (patient to staff):
- Immunisation against certain infectious diseases, eg hepatitis B, rubella, tuberculosis

- Wearing gloves

- Wearing eye protection glasses/visors/goggles

- Wearing appropriate clothing

- Handwashing

- Reducing aerosols in the surgery by using high-volume aspirators

- Using rubber dam for restorative procedures where appropriate

- Not re-sheathing needles

(c) This term means that all patients are treated equally with regards to cross-infection control, as normal measures should be of such a standard to prevent cross-infection. In other words, every patient is treated as though they were potentially infectious.

(d) Transmissible spongiform encephalopathy/Creutzfeldt–Jakob disease/new variant Creutzfeldt–Jakob disease

8.17 (a) Many instruments are sterilised in autoclaves; how does this differ from a hot air oven and what are the advantages of using an autoclave?

(b) Give one example regimen of how an autoclave achieves sterilisation.

(c) What methods are used to test that an autoclave is working effectively?

Answer 8.17

(a) Hot air ovens use dry heat to kill microorganisms and spores. They usually achieve temperatures of 160–180 °C, but at least an hour at this temperature is required for the procedure to be effective. Autoclaves use moist heat under pressure for sterilisation; this allows higher temperatures to be reached and so reduces the sterilisation time. Steam also contracts in volume during condensation, which increases penetration as well as liberates latent heat. Both these increase microbicidal activity.

(b) Any one of the following:
- 121–124°C for 15 minutes at 104 kPa
- 134–137°C for 3 minutes at 207 kPa

(c) Methods for testing autoclaves:
- Mechanical indicators on machine, eg temperature and pressure dials will tell you when appropriate settings have been reached.

- Process indicators are paper strips or liquids that change colour when they have been exposed to the appropriate settings. They will not prove that there are no pathogens remaining, just that the appropriate conditions were reached.

- Biological indicators actually prove that sterilisation has occurred. They contain bacterial spores which will lose their viability if the appropriate cycle conditions are reached. The indicators are removed from the autoclave and are cultured. If the spores are viable then the autoclave is not achieving sterilisation.

8.18 (a) What is the difference between sterilisation and disinfection?

(b) Name two items in a dental environment that are disinfected rather than sterilised.

(c) Chemicals are often used for disinfection. Name one other method of disinfection used in dentistry.

(d) Name three chemicals that may be used for disinfection in dentistry.

(e) What do you understand by the term antisepsis and when would it be used?

Answer 8.18

(a) Sterilisation is the removal of all living microorganisms and their pathogenic products whereas disinfection removes some of the microorganisms, usually the pathogenic ones.

(b) Any two of the following:
- Work surfaces in the surgery
- Light handles, chair arms, headrest, spittoon, etc.
- Patient safety glasses
- Impressions
- Collimating device

(c) Any one of the following:
- Heat (eg boiling)
- Physical (eg ultrasonics)

(d) Any three of the following:
- Alcohols
- Biguanides (eg chlorhexidine)
- Glutaraldehyde (this is banned in some areas)
- Chlorines
- Phenols

(e) Antisepsis is the application of a chemical agent externally on a live surface (eg skin or mucosa) to destroy organisms or to inhibit their growth. For example, preparing the skin prior to an operation or prior to taking a blood sample.

8.19 (a) What treatment should dirty but re-usable dental instruments undergo prior to sterilisation and why?

(b) How is this carried out?

(c) If items are not re-usable, they need to be disposed. How do you dispose of the following items?

- Suture needle

- Blood-stained gauze

- Waste amalgam

- Old record cards

(d) What do you understand by the term 'clinical waste'?

Answer 8.19

(a) All dirty instruments need to be cleaned prior to sterilisation to remove debris and organic material. This is because organic material (eg saliva and blood) remaining on instruments will increase the chances of survival of bacteria and can interfere with the sterilisation process. This cleaning process may be known as pre-sterilisation, reprocessing or decontamination.

(b) This process can be carried out manually by scrubbing them or using an ultrasonic bath, but ideally this cleaning process should be carried out with an automated and validated washer-disinfector. This is because washer-disinfectors have a disinfection stage that renders instruments safe for practice staff to handle and inspect.

(c) Methods of appropriate disposal:
- Suture needle — into a rigid sharps bin that will be incinerated
- Blood-stained gauze — in a clinical waste bag (usually yellow bag) that will be incinerated
- Amalgam — waste amalgam should be stored under liquid in a closed container until such time as it is collected by a specialised amalgam waste disposal service for disposal. It must not be put into clinical waste for incineration as mercury vapour will be produced.
- Old record cards — these contain confidential patient information so must not just be put in domestic waste. They must be disposed in such a way that patient information may not be read (by shredding or burning).

(d) Clinical waste is any waste that may be hazardous to any person coming into contact with it due to contamination with body fluids, eg blood and saliva.

8.20 (a) Clinical records are essential to the delivery of healthcare. What are such records?

(b) Give four examples of items used in dental treatment that would be classified as 'records'.

(c) Who has access to clinical records?

(d) For how long should dental records be kept?

(e) Computerised and manual patient records in dental practice are governed by which law in the UK and when was it introduced?

(f) Give three statements from this law.

Answer 8.20

(a) A medical record is any record which contains information relating to the physical or mental health or condition of an individual and has been made by or on behalf of a medical professional in connection with treatment of that individual.

(This definition is taken from the Health Professions Council.)

(b) Any four of the following:
- Clinical notes, whether handwritten or computerised
- Radiographs or other imaging records
- Photographs
- Study models
- Reports of investigations (eg laboratory reports)
- Correspondence about the patient
- Any recordings of the patient or conversations about the patient

(c) People who can access clinical records:
- Healthcare professionals involved in treating the patient
- The patient
- An insurance company paying for the treatment
- A court or the police (only when needed for investigation in a particular crime)

Note: confidential information may be shared if it is in the public interest, but you must be able to justify your decision.

(d) Length of time records should be kept:
- For adults — 11 years after the conclusion of treatment.
- For minors — until the age of 25 or 11 years since the conclusion of treatment, whichever is longer.

Note: This is not law but is what the defence organisations suggest as good practice.

(e) 1988 Data Protection Act

(f) Any three of the following:
- Data must be held securely.

- Data must be obtained fairly and for a specific and lawful purpose.

- Data must be used only for specific and lawful purposes.

- The patient should be able to access their data if they request it.

- Data should be adequate and relevant and not be excessive.

- Data should be disclosed only to certain individuals.

8.21 (a) Patients need to give consent for dental treatment. List five conditions that must be fulfilled for consent to be described as informed when treating an adult.

(b) What types of informed consent are there? Explain what they are.

(c) For which types of treatment is consent needed?

(d) When must a patient sign a consent form?

Answer 8.21

(a) Five conditions that must be fulfilled for consent:
- Patient aged over 16 years (unless they are Gillick/Fraser competent).
- Consent must be freely given.
- All risks and benefits must be explained to patient and the patient must understand them.
- All treatment options must be given to the patient.
- The patient must be able to understand and give consent (ie competent).

(b) Types of consent:
- Implied consent — the patient's actions imply that they are happy for the treatment to commence. For example, a patient sitting in the dental chair and opening their mouth for an examination.
- Verbal consent — the treatment is explained to the patient and the patient agrees verbally to it.
- Written consent — the patient signs a form to say that they agree to the treatment being carried out. It is usually reserved for conditions when the patient's level of consciousness will be altered and they do not have the capacity to terminate the treatment if they wanted to.

(c) All types of treatment require consent, otherwise it is classified as assault.

(d) Procedures in which consciousness is altered — intravenous sedation and general anaesthesia. It is also useful to ask patients to sign a consent form when there is a risk of serious complications, eg damage to the inferior dental or lingual nerve during surgical removal of lower third molars.

8.22 (a) What does the abbreviation GDC stand for and what is the principal role of this body?

(b) What are the statutory responsibilities of the GDC?

(c) How much time for continuing professional development (CPD) is required by the GDC? What topics do they strongly recommend you include in that CPD?

(d) Who must be registered with the GDC?

Answer 8.22

(a) General Dental Council. The GDC is the regulatory body of the dental profession and professions complementary to dentistry. The principal role is protecting the public.

(b) Statutory responsibilities of the GDC:

- To promote, at all stages, high standards of education in all aspects of dentistry.

- To promote high standards of professional conduct, performance and practice among persons registered under the Dentist Act 1984.

(c) The GDC requires dentists to do 250 hours of CPD in a 5-year cycle. Within that, 75 hours must be verifiable CPD. They strongly recommend that 10 hours should be dedicated to medical emergencies, 5 hours to disinfection and decontamination and 5 hours to radiographs and radiation protection. They also recommend that the early detection of oral cancer, legal and ethical issues, and handling complaints be covered in every cycle.

(d) All dentists, clinical dental technicians, dental nurses, dental hygenists, dental technicians, dental therapists and orthodontic therapists must register with the GDC.

8.23 (a) What do you understand by the term 'dental negligence'?

    (b) Claims of negligence have to be made within certain time limits. What are these limits?

    (c) Patients have the right to complain about aspects of their treatment. If a patient wishes to complain about treatment in a dental practice how should the process be conducted?

Answer 8.23

(a) This term means the dentist had a duty of care that was breached and that damage resulted from that breach of care.

(b) Within 3 years from the date of the knowledge of the negligence occurring or 6 years from the incident occurring or within 6 years of reaching the age of majority if the negligence occurred in a minor.

(c) Complaints procedure:

1   A copy of the written complaints procedure must be available for patients and a copy should be given to the patient when you acknowledge their complaint.

2   Send an acknowledgement of complaint within 3 working days.

3   Contact your dental defence organisation.

4   Respond in writing or by telephone as soon as possible, but no later than 10 working days.

5   If more time is needed to investigate the complaint you should inform the patient of this in your acknowledgment.

6   Regularly update your patient with your progress in investigating the complaint, at least every 10 working days.

7   Offer an apology and practical solution.

8   If the patient is not satisfied tell them about the NHS complaints procedures (or the Dental Complaints Service for private patients).

9   Patients have the right to appeal to their primary care trust for an independent review panel, or to the Healthcare Commission, and if not satisfied they can approach the NHS Ombudsman.

8.24 (a) What do you understand by the term 'clinical audit'?

(b) What are the stages of an audit cycle?

(c) Dental professionals have a duty of care to their patients and must put patient's interests first. In what circumstances would you have a responsibility to raise any concern you have that patients might be at risk?

Answer 8.24

(a) This is the systematic critical analysis of the quality of clinical care, including procedures used for diagnosis and treatment, use of resources and patient outcome.

(b) Stages of an audit cycle:

   1 Identify the procedure or treatment method that is to be audited.

   2 Set the standards.

   3 Measure the performance against the standard that you have set.

   4 Analyse the results. If the standard has not been reached then clarify the problem and determine what changes need to be introduced to achieve the standard.

   5 Implement change.

   6 Re-measure the performance following implementation against the standard.

(c) If you believed patients might be at risk because:

   • Of the health, behaviour or professional performance of a colleague or employer

   • Of any aspect of the clinical environment

   • Or if you have been asked to carry out any action that you believe conflicts with your duty to put patients' interests first

8.25   You are suturing an extraction socket and you accidentally prick yourself with the suture needle (needlestick injury). How should you now proceed?

Answer 8.25

1 Stop what you are doing.

2 Encourage the wound to bleed.

3 Wash it under running water and use a detergent if available but do not scrub.

4 Cover with waterproof plaster.

5 A risk assessment of the patient needs to be carried out — this is usually done by another person so as to eliminate a conflict of interest. The status of the patient with respect to transmissible diseases needs to be assessed; usually the patient is tested for hepatitis B and C and human immunodeficiency virus (HIV) by a blood test after the risk assessment.

6 Your hepatitis B status should be assessed. As the needle is not a hollow-bore needle and you would have been wearing gloves the risk is lower.

7 The incident should be recorded in an incident book.

8 Ensure that the patient's treatment is completed.

9 If there is any cause for concern you should liaise with your local point of contact for accidental body fluid exposures. This may be your occupational health department/accident and emergency department/microbiologist/physician, depending on where you work.

Note: local policies may differ slightly.

8.26 (a) What does IR(ME)R stand for, and when did these regulations come into force.

(b) According to IR(ME)R what is the role of the following people and who may undertake these roles?

(i)   Referrer

(ii)   Practitioner

(iii)   Operator

(iv)   Employer

Answer 8.26

(a) IR(ME)R stands for Ionising Radiation (Medical Exposure) Regulations and they came into force in 2000.

(b) Description of the roles:
  (i) A referrer is responsible for supplying the practitioner with sufficient information to justify the radiograph being taken. They are usually a dentist or doctor but other healthcare professionals with appropriate training may be entitled to refer patients for radiographs.

  (ii) A practitioner justifies that the radiograph is necessary and that the benefits outweigh the risks. They are usually a dentist or doctor although other healthcare professionals who are entitled to take responsibility may assume the role of practitioner.

  (iii) An operator is any person who carries out part or all of the tasks associated with taking the radiograph including actually taking the radiograph. They must be adequately trained and are usually dentists or dental nurses, hygienists and therapists who have undergone adequate training.

  (iv) An employer or legal person is the person with legal responsibility for a radiological installation. They must ensure that the regulations are enforced and that good practice is followed. They are usually the practice owner.

Index